Other monographs in the series, Major Problems in Clinical Surgery:

EXENTERATIVE SURGERY OF THE PELVIS

John S. Spratt, Jr., M.S.P.H., M.D.

Director, Cancer Research Center, Columbia, Missouri;
Chief Surgeon, Ellis Fischel State Cancer Hospital,
Columbia, Missouri and Lecturer in Surgery,
Washington University School of Medicine, St. Louis, Missouri

Harvey R. Butcher, Jr., M.D.

Professor of Surgery, Washington University School of Medicine,
St. Louis, Missouri and Assistant Surgeon,
Barnes Hospital, St. Louis, Missouri

Eugene M. Bricker, M.D.

Clinical Professor of Surgery, Washington University School
of Medicine, St. Louis, Missouri and Associate Surgeon,
Barnes Hospital, St. Louis, Missouri

Volume XII in the Series

**MAJOR PROBLEMS IN
CLINICAL SURGERY**

J. ENGLEBERT DUNPHY, M.D.
Consulting Editor

W. B. Saunders Company, Philadelphia, London, Toronto, 1973

W. B. Saunders Company: West Washington Square
Philadelphia, Pa.   19105

12 Dyott Street
London, WC1A   1DB

833 Oxford Street
Toronto 18, Ontario

Exenterative Surgery of the Pelvis   ISBN   0-7216-8523-4

Print No: 9   8   7   6   5   4   3   2   1

Foreword

Extended surgery for advanced cancer of the pelvis has become an accepted and very appropriate operation in selected cases. In this volume Dr. John Spratt and his colleagues present their experience of 30 years with this procedure.

The precise indications for operation, the surgical technique, the prevention and management of complications and, most important of all, the total care of the patient are described in detail. The great benefit of the operation, in those situations in which its use is clearly indicated, is thoroughly documented. By exercising care in the selection of patients for this operation and applying the principles presented in this book, operative mortality can be kept to a minimum.

The value of this book goes far beyond the application of basic principles to pelvic exenteration. All surgeons who have occasion to operate on the pelvic viscera will profit from this important review. Urologists, gynecologists and general surgeons, as well as oncologic surgeons, will find this an important reference work. There is no telling when a particular tumor may require more extended exposure and dissection than is anticipated. A familiarity with the basic principles and the details of surgical technique outlined in detail here will prove of inestimable value to every surgeon who undertakes major pelvic operations.

The authors are to be congratulated for the thoroughness of this study based largely on their own extensive experience.

J. ENGLEBERT DUNPHY

Foreword

Few significant advances in surgery or in other science, for that matter, develop *de novo*. Careful observation of the natural behavior of various types of pelvic cancer by surgeons intimately familiar with the complexities of the anatomy of the pelvic fascia has permitted evolution of the operation now known as pelvic exenteration. The opportunity, then, for such a major therapeutic advance was presented simultaneously to a number of surgeons interested in treatment of pelvic cancers. Many surgeons made contributions toward the complete removal of these locally recurrent cancers, but it remained for an unusually skilled team of surgeons to perfect the operation, not only removing the necessary pelvic tissue but also developing far better reconstructive procedures than had been used before.

The patients who comprise this study were seen at the Ellis Fischel State Cancer Hospital in Columbia, Missouri, and at Barnes Hospital, Saint Louis, Missouri, some one hundred miles apart, yet the surgeons, anatomists and pathologists whose contributions to the understanding of locally recurrent pelvic cancer have made these advances possible have worked closely together the past quarter century as a team of clinical scientists. That so many of these patients were spared the misery of pain accompanying uncontrolled recurrent disease and were permitted many productive years after operation is due to the skill and imagination of Drs. Eugene Bricker, Harvey Butcher and John Spratt. The fact that each surgeon continued his careful observation of each patient permitted the remarkably complete follow-up data described in this volume.

Thus, a prepared mind, a creative imagination, a skilled hand and a dedication to patient care are the essential ingredients. Each of the authors of this monograph embody this splendid combination.

WALTER F. BALLINGER, M.D.

Preface

The purpose of this monograph is to record the historical, technical and end result experience of the authors in the surgical management of advanced pelvic neoplasms by exenterative surgery of the pelvis. The experience extends from 1940 to the present at two hospitals: the Ellis Fischel State Cancer Hospital (EFSCH) in Columbia, Missouri, and the Barnes Hospital in Saint Louis, Missouri. The experience would not have been possible without the numerous general surgical residents and the hospital staffs who participated in patient care. Particular appreciation is expressed to Dr. Carlos Perez-Mesa, Dr. R. E. Johnson and their associates at EFSCH and Dr. L. V. Ackerman at Barnes Hospital for the detailed anatomical pathological studies performed on the surgical specimens. These studies have made a vital contribution to our understanding of the pathology of advanced pelvic neoplasms.

The patients reported in the end results studies were all seen by one of the authors. They were referred because they had neoplasms that had extended beyond the organ of origin and were no longer controllable by organocentric surgery or because their cancers had persisted or recurred in the pelvis after radiotherapy or an organocentric procedure that inadequately removed the extraorgan extensions of the neoplasms. Consequently, the surgical technology has been developed to manage the unique problems presented by the neoplasms. The ablative surgical techniques involve multiorgan resection by fascial plane dissection in the pelvis. The reconstructive techniques have evolved to restore the vital function of the removed viscera. The techniques of pre- and postoperative care unique to the operations are described.

Since the data and techniques in this monograph deal largely with the personal experience of the authors, the work is neither comprehensive from the bibliographical standpoint nor is it intended to provide complete information on the routine pre- and postoperative aspects of patient care. The presumption is made that any surgeon undertaking pelvic exenterations will already be well trained and will need collateral information to augment his basic knowledge. This attitude affects both the organization and content of the book.

The chapters include a historical résumé by the developer of many of the basic surgical techniques (EMB). The chapter on anatomy draws its content almost entirely from Uhlenhuth and attempts to give the reader an appreciation of the fascial anatomy of the pelvis.[1] Exenterative surgery in the pelvis, just as regional ablative surgery for cancer in other areas of the body, involves fascial plane dissection. The technique of fascial plane dissection has features in common in all body regions — the main variable is the fascial anatomy itself. The anatomical nomenclature was updated from Uhlenhuth's work by Daniel E. Overack, Ph.D., Assistant Professor of Anatomy at the University of Missouri School of Medicine in Columbia, Missouri.

The chapters covering indications, contraindications, end results, surgical technique, and pre- and postoperative care were compiled by Drs. Spratt and Butcher and edited by Dr. Bricker. The follow-up of the EFSCH cases was compiled by Miriam G. Hoag, Director of Social Service, and Freda M. Tarr, Supervisor of Medical Records. In both the EFSCH and Barnes the follow-up on all cases was 100 per cent. The computer programs for life tables on the EFSCH cases were developed by the biomathematics unit of the Cancer Research Center (CRC) under Dr. F. R. Watson and Mr. Richard LeDuc. Miss Cynthia Cunningham and Mrs. Barbara Willenberg provided invaluable editing and stenographic contributions. Mrs. Linda Wilson and Miss Libby Forbis contributed to the photography and graphic illustrations, respectively. Mrs. Bonnie Gordon, R.N., operating room supervisor, contributed invaluable assistance in compiling the chapter on surgical instruments used in pelvic exenteration. Mrs. Ruth C. Wakerlin, Chief, Medical Illustrations, Section of Medical Educational Services, University Medical Center, University of Missouri, Columbia, Missouri, prepared the illustrations for the surgical techniques used in constructing an ileal bladder.

The chapters on surgical technique were originally written in SURTRAN.[2] SURTRAN clarifies and facilitates the written description of a surgical technique. Each step of the technique is written down in a direct positive voice sentence. These are then transferred to IBM cards, and a sequential printout is made for review. Both the description and the sequence of steps are checked against an actual surgical operation to avoid errors that might be attributable to the surgeon's recollection of his technique. Originally, it had been our

---

[1]Uhlenhuth, E.: Problems in the Anatomy of the Pelvis, An Atlas. Philadelphia, J. B. Lippincott Company, 1953.

[2]Cook, G. B., and Watson, F. R.: SURTRAN, Linear graphing of surgical decisions and activities. J. Surg. Res., 9:361, 1969.

intent to publish the actual SURTRAN card printouts. However, in testing the printouts against the written paragraph, the paragraph was more acceptable to most readers. Consequently, the SURTRAN for the various surgical subroutines used in exenterative surgery of the pelvis has been edited into conventional paragraphs. As these surgical descriptions are read, the information in the anatomy chapter should be kept in mind. The authors have relied on the combination of operative description and the anatomical drawings as a substitute for extensive drawings of surgical technique.

JOHN S. SPRATT, JR.

HARVEY R. BUTCHER, JR.

EUGENE M. BRICKER

Contents

xi

Chapter One

HISTORY

The possibility of applying extended surgery to selected advanced pelvic cancers appears to have occurred to surgeons in three areas of the North American continent at roughly the same time in the early 1940's. At the Ellis Fischel State Cancer Hospital (EFSCH) in 1940 and 1941 it was recognized that there were certain variants of cancer of the colon that might grow to involve contiguous viscera without being disseminated through the lymphatic or blood stream. Such lesions of the abdominal colon, when recognized, were removed totally by multiple visceral resections. The same tumor characteristics were recognized in the pelvic colon and rectum, but the problem of the advanced lesion in this area was complicated by the necessity for sacrifice of the lower urinary tract. A small group of patients were operated upon for a huge carcinoma of the prostate mistaken for a carcinoma of the rectum. The ureters in one of the patients were transferred to an isolated segment of the sigmoid colon which was brought out on the same side of the abdomen as the terminal colostomy. Although this method of urinary diversion left much to be desired, the patient got along quite well until he died of disseminated bone metastases approximately 18 months after operation. Surgical cements and glued-on appliances were not known to us at that time. These early excursions into ultra-radical pelvic surgery at the EFSCH were interrupted by World War II, and the cases were never reported.

In 1948 Brunschwig published the first paper on the subject, reporting his results in the treatment of advanced carcinoma of the cervix extending back over the preceding two years. In 1950 Appleby, of Canada, reported the results of "proctocystectomy" in a group of patients with advanced carcinoma of the rectum, one of whom was a seven-year survivor, having been operated upon in 1943. Apparently

1

Appleby was the first to carry the operation to completion with enough success to justify publication. Urinary diversion in his patients, as well as in Brunschwig's patients, was by ureterocolic anastomosis, leaving the patient with a "wet colostomy." It was Brunschwig's paper in 1948 that gave numerical significance to the possibilities of the operation, since the number of patients with advanced or recurrent carcinoma of the cervix was so much greater than the occasional patient with carcinoma of the rectum or rectosigmoid that might require exenteration for control.

After World War II, the problem was pursued further at Barnes Hospital in Saint Louis. At this time (1946) attention was still confined to patients with advanced carcinoma of the rectum. The pathological and anatomical justification for the operation seemed obvious. The major remaining unsolved problem concerned the method of urinary diversion after removal of the rectum. Attention was still focused on this facet of the problem with really no satisfactory solution until 1950 when the concept of using an ileal conduit evolved. It was also in 1950 that operations on recurrent carcinoma of the cervix were started at Barnes Hospital (by E.M.B.) after urging from Dr. A. N. Arneson of the Department of Gynecology at Washington University School of Medicine. Prior to this time, one of us (E.M.B.) had doubted the biological suitability of advanced or recurrent carcinoma of the cervix for exenteration. Time has proved that carcinoma of the cervix does have biological characteristics making it suitable for extended surgery in selected cases; after 1950 an increasing number of surgeons, general surgeons and gynecologists became interested in exenterative surgery for advanced pelvic cancers, and the number of contributors to the literature of this subject grew to become international in scope (Bricker, 1954 and 1951; Brunschwig, 1965, 1964 and 1966; Dargent; Douglas; Ingersoll; Ingiulla; Kiselow; Mattingly; Parsons, 1954 and 1964; Rutledge; Schmitz; and Smith).

These reports are concerned predominantly with carcinoma of the cervix, and there seems to be general agreement on the following points: (1) the surgery is justified for selected lesions on the basis of pathological and biological characteristics, (2) the mortality and morbidity rates can be reasonable and acceptable, (3) the five-year survival rate can be gratifying and even better than the rates for several other malignancies operated upon in a more "operable" stage, (4) rehabilitation to a useful and healthful existence is to be expected if the disease is controlled and (5) without exenterative removal of these cancers the patient has a protracted, painful and miserable terminal course which is quite costly from the standpoint of terminal nursing care.

Diversion of urinary excretion has been a concomitant and corollary problem with the other features of pelvic exenteration. For several reasons, our own research in this area remained completely clinical and no laboratory experimentation was resorted to until after the ileal segment conduit was in regular use. It was at this point that the absorption of urinary constituents from the ileal segment was studied by Eiseman, and the emptying power of the segments and their function as a conduit was reported by Klinge. This aggressive application of a new procedure without prior laboratory investigation seemed perfectly justified for the following reasons: (1) the primary consideration in the patients for whom urinary diversion was done was the cure of cancer too far advanced to permit successful control with a lesser surgical procedure, (2) ureterointestinal (sigmoidal) anastomoses had been done for years, and whether the anastomosis was done to the intact intestinal tract or to an isolated segment seemed inconsequential, and (3) the possible differences between a short segment of terminal ileum and segment of the colon or the intact colon seemed not enough to demand delay in the application of the new procedure.

The advent of the watertight ileostomy appliances was a most important development in the search for a solution to urinary diversion. It is interesting that, from the first, our efforts were aimed at fashioning some type of intra-abdominal receptacle for the urine which was to be under the voluntary control of the patient. Brunschwig and Appleby, on the other hand, adopted the concept of the "wet colostomy" in their early cases. Our first attempts to develop an intra-abdominal receptacle were made at EFSCH in 1940 when a short segment of sigmoid colon was used. Following the war, we went through a period of using terminal ileum and cecum which was to be under voluntary control of the patient through use of a catheter (Bricker and Eiseman, 1950). The results of these attempts were unsatisfactory because patients were still unable to keep themselves clean, dry and odor-free. Gilchrist and Merricks used cecum in much the same manner with results they found to be more satisfactory.

It was at this stage (1949) that Dr. Heinz Haffner, when operating upon a patient at Saint Louis City Hospital, found it impossible to use the cecum as a receptacle for the ureters, as was our current custom. Instead he transplanted the ureters to an isolated segment of terminal ileum and brought the open end out through the abdominal wall. Since this patient did not survive to leave the hospital, the significance of the ileal segment as a conduit could not be appreciated, though the operation was essentially the same type we started doing deliberately a few months later.

It was just at this time that surgical cements and improved external appliances were coming into general use in the management of ileostomies following colectomy. These bags were applied to our leaking and unsatisfactory cecal pouches and served to relieve the patient immediately of the unpleasant consequences of an inadequately controlled urinary fistula. In view of this development, the logical next step was to forgo all efforts at making an intra-abdominal reservoir and simply to provide a conduit for the urine from both ureters to a convenient location on the abdominal wall. A segment of terminal ileum seemed to be the simplest way to accomplish this end, and our first planned ileal conduit operations were done in 1950 (Bricker, 1950). The immediate results were so gratifying that it has been continued ever since. From the standpoint of technical simplicity and operating time, it has been found to be practical to combine the procedure with pelvic exenteration. Also, in comparison with our previous experiences, the patients were so dry and comfortable that any objection on our part to accepting an external appliance as a solution was dispelled.

This sporadic evolution of the ileal conduit was a very fortunate occurrence in that it was an acceptable solution for one of the most vexing problems associated with pelvic exenteration. The door was opened to the application of this type of surgery to many people who might receive benefit from it. Although some surgeons continued to use the "wet colostomy," the ileal segment operation won an increasing following as the years progressed, and at the present time it is the most satisfactory and frequently used means of urinary diversion for both benign and malignant lesions. The procedure is not without complications, as is attested to by reported clinical studies; however, it has served us well and with a few minor technical alterations has remained our preferred means of substituting for the urinary bladder. Recent comprehensive surveys of the results of the ileal conduit operation included those of Jaffe, Small, Harbach, Cordonnier, Butcher, and Long.

As is frequently the case, it was learned subsequent to our initial publication (Bricker, 1950) on the subject of ileal segment urinary diversion that the idea was really not new. Mersheimer and Kolarsick (1950, 1951) had used ileal segments in a similar fashion in dogs at the same time we started doing the operation in humans. It was also discovered that Seiffert, a German surgeon, had used a jejunal segment in a similar manner and had published the result in 1935. In 1916 Blair had transplanted the ureters to the bypassed terminal ileum which drained through the ileocecal valve into the intact colon. Tizzoni and Foggi in 1888 experimentally used a segment of small intestine to receive the ureters and placed the distal end of the segment under control of the vesical sphincter (Hinmann). In 1911 Cuneo used a segment of bowel in a similar fashion with the end being brought out through the anal sphincter (Hinmann). All of these attempts, with the exception of that of Seiffert, aimed at using a bowel segment as an internal conduit to place release of urine under some type of voluntary control.

REFERENCES

Appleby, L. H.: Proctocystectomy; management of colostomy with ureteral transplants. Am. J. Surg., 79:57, 1950.

Blair, V. P.: Implantation of the trigonum into the segregated lower end of the ileum. Surg. Gynecol. Obstet., 22:352, 1916.

Bricker, E. M.: Bladder substitution after pelvic evisceration. Surg. Clin. North Am., 30:1511, 1950.

Bricker, E. M.: Total exenteration of the pelvic organs. In Meigs, J. V. (ed.): Surgical Treatment of Cancer of the Cervix. New York, Grune & Stratton, Inc., 1954, pp. 349–374.

Bricker, E. M., and Eiseman, B.: Bladder reconstruction from cecum and ascending colon following resection of pelvic viscera. Ann. Surg., 132:77, 1950.

Bricker, E. M., and Eiseman, B.: Electrolyte absorption following bilateral ureteroenterostomy into an isolated intestinal segment. Ann. Surg., 136:751, 1952.

Bricker, E. M., and Klinge, F. W.: The evacuation of urine by ileal segments in man. Ann. Surg., 137:36, 1953.

Bricker, E. M., and Modlin, J.: The role of pelvic evisceration in surgery. Surgery, 30:76, 1951.

Brunschwig, A.: Complete excision of pelvic viscera for advanced carcinoma. Cancer, 1:177, 1948.

Brunschwig, A.: What are the indications and results of pelvic exenteration? J.A.M.A., 194:274, 1965.

Brunschwig, A., and Barber, H. R. K.: Extended pelvic exenteration for advanced carcinoma of the cervix. Cancer, 17:1267, 1964.

Brunschwig, A., and Barber, H. R. K.: Surgical treatment of carcinoma of the cervix. Obstet. Gynecol., 27:21, 1966.

Butcher, H. R., Jr., Sugg, W. L., McAfee, C. A., and Bricker, E. M.: Ileal conduit method of ureteral urinary diversion. Ann. Surg., 156:682, 1962.

Cordonnier, J. J.: Surgery of the ureters and urinary conduits. In Campbell, M. F. (ed.): Urology. Vol. 3. Philadelphia, W. B. Saunders Company, 1963, pp. 2419–2466.

Dargent, M., Mayer, M., and Colon, J.: Les limites et les indications de l'exentération pelvienne pour cancer gynécologique en phase avancée. C. R. Soc. Franc. Gynecol., 27:293, 1957.

Douglas, R. G., and Sweeney, W. J.: Exenteration operation in treatment of advanced pelvic cancer. Am. J. Obstet. Gynecol., 73:1169, 1957.

Gilchrist, R. K., and Merricks, J. W.: Construction of a substitute bladder and urethra. Surg. Clin. North Am., 36:1, 1956.

Harbach, L. B., Hall, R. L., Cockett, A. T. K., Kaufman, J. J., Martin, D. C., Mims, M. M., and Goodwin, W. E.: Ileal loop cutaneous urinary diversion: a critical review. J. Urol., 105:511, 1971.

Hinman, F., and Weyrauch, H. M., Jr.: A critical study of the different principles of surgery which have been used in ureterointestinal implantation. Int. Abstr. Surg., 64:313, 1937.

Ingersoll, F., and Ulfelder, H.: Pelvic exenteration for carcinoma of the cervix. N. Engl. J. Med., 274:648, 1966.

Ingiulla, W., and Cosmi, E. V.: Pelvic exenteration for advanced carcinoma of the cervix. Some reflections on 241 cases. Am. J. Obstet. Gynecol., 99:1083, 1967.

Jaffe, B. M., Bricker, E. M., and Butcher, H. R., Jr.: Surgical complications of ileal segment urinary diversion. Ann. Surg., 167:367, 1968.

Kiselow, M., Butcher, H. R., Jr., and Bricker, E. M.: Results of the radical surgical treatment of advanced pelvic cancer: a fifteen-year study. Ann. Surg., 166:428, 1967.

Long, R. T. L., Grummon, R. A., Spratt, J. S., Jr., and Perez-Mesa, C.: Carcinoma of the urinary bladder (comparison with radical, simple and partial cystectomy and intravesical formalin). Cancer, 29:98, 1972.

Mattingly, R. F.: Total pelvic exenteration. Clin. Obstet. Gynecol., 8:705, 1965.

Mersheimer, W. L., Kolarsick, A. J., and Kammandel, H.: Implantation of ureters into completely isolated loops of small intestine. Proc. Soc. Exp. Biol. Med., 76:1970, 1951.

Mersheimer, W. L., Kolarsick, A. J., and Kammandel, H.: Method for construction of artificial urinary bladder by implantation of ureters into completely or partially excluded segments of small intestines. Bull. N.Y. Med. Coll., *13*:71, 1950.

Parsons, L.: Total exenteration of the pelvic organs. *In* Meigs, J. V. (ed.): Surgical Treatment of Cancer of the Cervix. New York, Grune & Stratton, Inc., 1954, pp. 322–348.

Parsons, L., and Friedell, G. H.: Radical surgical treatment of carcinoma of the cervix. Proc. Natl. Cancer Conf., 5:241, 1964.

Rutledge, F. N., and Burns, B. C.: Pelvic exenteration. Am. J. Obstet. Gynecol., *91*:692, 1965.

Schmitz, H. E., Schmitz, R. L., Smith, C. J., and Molitor, J. J.: The technique of synchronous (two team) abdominoperineal pelvic exenteration. Surg. Gynecol. Obstet., *108*:351, 1959.

Seiffert, L.: Die "Darm-Siphonblase." Arch. Klin. Chir., *183*:569, 1935.

Small, M. P., Boyarsky, S., and Glenn, J. F.: Clinical and experimental evaluation of ileal segment urinary diversion. Am. J. Surg., *115*:782, 1968.

Smith, R. R., Ketcham, A. S., and Thomas, L. B.: Carcinoma of uterine cervix. Cancer, *16*:1105, 1963.

Chapter Two

SURGICAL ANATOMY

The key to most cancer surgery is fascial plane dissection. All viscera giving rise to cancer, whether they be hollow or parenchymatous, have an important relationship to the regional fascial anatomy. The viscus, its afferent lymphatics and the first order lymph nodes receiving the affluent lymph usually lie within an identifiable sheet of deep fascia. Design of the surgical resection requires a clear understanding of this fascial envelope. The fascial envelope and the cancerous viscus must be resected en bloc if the operation is to be curative for those cancers that grow by direct extension beyond their viscus of origin or metastasize to first order lymph nodes. In no region of the body are these statements more certain than in the pelvis. Consequently, a discussion of these fascial relations and their significance to the cancer surgeon during the course of his dissection is primary in a consideration of the surgical anatomy.

The visceral layer of pelvic fascia lies directly adjacent the hollow pelvic organs. Cancers with protuberant nonmetastasizing growth, such as low-grade papillomas in the bladder and polypoid and villous carcinomas of the rectum, permit curative surgery by dissecting immediately adjacent to the viscus, i.e., adjacent its visceral fascia. If, however, the cancer has invaded into the deeper layers of the viscus, the depth of invasion only occasionally penetrates more than half of the greatest chordal dimensions of the primary cancer. An ulcerated invasive bladder or rectal cancer 1 cm. in its greatest chordal dimension often extends to a depth of 5 mm. If an infiltrating cancer has a surface diameter more than twice the thickness of a viscus, there is

Figure 2-1 1, Rectum; 2, parietal fascia over the coccygeus muscle; 3, superior surface of bladder covered by fascial capsule of bladder; 4, cervical portion of uterus; 5, external iliac vessels; 6, internal iliac artery; 7, internal iliac vein; 8, lateral wing of pelvic sheath (separated from bladder by a dorsoventral incision); 9, hypogastric plexus; 10, dorsal wall of peritoneal rectovaginal pouch (with rectovaginal septum attached to the bottom of the pouch); 11, sacral sympathetic trunk; 12, sympathetic branches from first and second sympathetic ganglion to hypogastric plexus; 13, parasympathetic branches from third, fourth and fifth sacral nerves; 14, presacral wing of pelvic sheath; 18, ureter in inferior hypogastric wing of visceral fascia; 25 and 25′, rubber tube through concave fascia from lateral compartment retropubic space into presacral space; 26 and 26′, rubber tube through hole in the bottom of retropubic space into the presacral space.

Description: This figure shows the space dorsal to the presacral wing of the pelvic sheath and the relation of the presacral wing of visceral fascia to the rectum. For this purpose, the bladder and lateral wing (8) have been replaced into their normal position, the cervix and vagina (4) have been returned to their normal position, the remaining peritoneum of the rectouterine pouch (10) has been pulled forward over the uterus and the presacral wing has been raised from the dorsal pelvic wall and reflected forward.

Laterally the presacral wing is attached to the internal iliac artery (6) and internal iliac vein (7) (where it becomes continuous with the medial leaf of the dorsal wing and lateral wing). The reflection of the presacral wing permits a view into the presacral (i.e., retrorectal) space and exposes the dorsal wall of this space. It now becomes evident that behind the presacral wing or visceral fascia there is located still another fascia, the parietal fascia, which lines the pelvic surfaces of the coccygeus muscle (2) and, higher up, of the pyriformis muscle. In this space are found the visceral nerves and among them, in the first place, the *inferior hypogastric plexus* (9). This has been pulled away from the pelvic wall; normally it represents the most medial structure among all the structures which take a craniocaudal course; it runs at a more medial course than the ureter which is next to it laterally. The sympathetic trunk (11) with its ganglia, of which the uppermost is the first sacral ganglion, is also visible; sympathetic branches (12) from the first and second ganglia are seen to join the hypogastric plexus. And finally, the parasympathetic branches (13), which have pierced the parietal fascia and are arising in this subject from the third, fourth and fifth sacral nerves, are seen passing forward into the presacral wing of the hypogastric sheath. All these nerves (hypogastric as well as parasympathetic) pierce the presacral wing to enter into the space formed between a dorsal leaf and a ventral leaf of this wing; in this space is located the pelvic plexus which is joined by these nerves. In the normal pelvis, before dissection, all these nerves take a lateral course and are apposed to the wall of the pelvis; in the dissected specimen illustrated in this figure they seem to have a more dorsoventral course because they have been pulled away from the wall with the presacral fascia to which they are attached. The plexus has frontal extension; laterally it lies about at the level of the ischial spine from where it extends medially and ventrally and comes to lie with its medial boundary just dorsal to the lateral cervical ligament.

It is possible now to define the boundaries of the presacral space. Dorsally it is bounded by the parietal fascia of the coccygeus and pyriformis, ventrally by the presacral wing of the pelvic sheath and laterally it is closed by attachment of the latter wing to the internal iliac vessels. In the undisturbed pelvis there is no connection between this space and any of the other fascial spaces; in particular, this space is separated from the lateral compartment of the retropubic space by the dorsal wing of the pelvic sheath and by the pelvic fascia. From the retropubic space, however, access can be created to the presacral space in the manner shown by the markers of rubber tubing (25 and 26). It will be noticed that the more cranial of these rubber tubings (25′) was put through the concave fascia just caudal to the inferior vesical arch and arrives in the presacral space just caudal to the parasympathetic nerves; if a finger is pushed through the concave fascia, it usually hits against these nerves.

It is of importance to consider the relationship which exists between the presacral space on the one hand and the rectovaginal and vesicovaginal spaces on the other hand. If a probe is pushed through the passageway indicated by the rubber tubing (26′ and 26), it will always come out in the lateral compartment of the cave of Retzius (retropubic space) passing between the presacral fascia and the parietal fascia lining the coccygeus and levator ani and lateral to the attachments of the lateral margins of the rectovaginal septum and of the fascial wing of the vagina. If it is desired to create a passage between the presacral and rectovaginal spaces, it is necessary to push the probe medially as soon as it arrives at the level of the vagina and to perforate both the presacral fascia and the fascial wing which attaches the vagina to the presacral fascia.

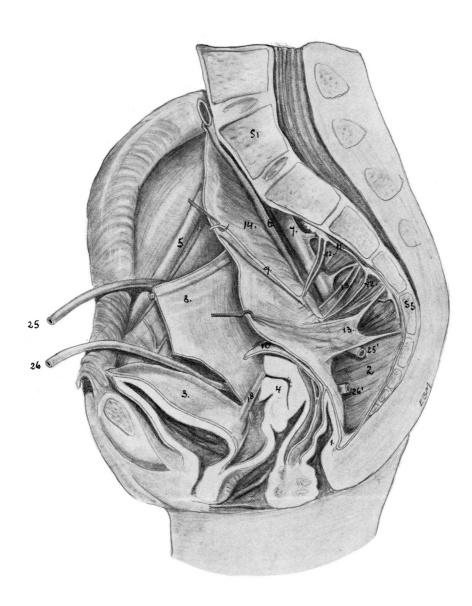

Figure 2–1. *See opposite page for legend.*

high probability that it continues through the visceral fascia encompassing the viscus. When this occurs the cancer extends directly into the fatty areolar tissue lying between the visceral and parietal layers of fascia. In this fatty areolar tissue are the afferent lymphatics, lymph nodes and blood vessels. The nerves to the pelvic viscera are primarily autonomic and follow the arteries to the viscera. Only one somatic nerve of importance, the obturator nerve, actually lies on the visceral side of the parietal layer of pelvic fascia. Since the nerve is immediately adjacent to the fascia, the fascia can generally be incised over the nerve, separating the nerve from the central pelvic tissue mass without exposing neoplasm. Occasionally, the proximity of cancer necessitates the sacrifice of this nerve to insure an adequate margin around the neoplasm. Transection of the obturator nerve on one side leaves a tolerable disability. When it is resected on both sides, the disability is more significant. The patient with bilateral transection can walk but cannot adduct the thighs voluntarily.

The anatomy of the pelvis has to be viewed in nonorganocentric perspective by a surgeon performing a pelvic exenteration. Exenteration of the pelvis involves fascial plane dissection with total removal of all viscera lying between the fascial planes enveloped by the dissection. The removal of various organs lying within the enveloping fascia is the secondary objective of the surgery. The primary objective is the en bloc removal of cancer that has extended beyond the organ of origin.

In this view, exenterative surgery of the pelvis has many characteristics in common with other cancer operations requiring extensive fascial plane dissection. The anatomical and surgical literature contains little detailed writing on the fascial anatomy of the pelvis. However, search brought forth the meticulous work of Eduard Uhlenhuth, entitled *Problems in the Anatomy of the Pelvis, An Atlas,* published in 1953. Dr. Uhlenhuth was professor of anatomy at the University of Maryland. He was succeeded on his retirement by Professor Frank H. J. Figge, a former student (Figge, 1962 and 1971).

Professor Uhlenhuth was an accomplished and productive anatomist when his wife developed carcinoma of the urinary bladder. In reviewing her problem with one of the senior American urologists he became aware of the fact that surgeons really knew very little about the anatomy of the human pelvis. Indeed, most gross anatomy texts still deal with this complicated region in a very superficial manner. Uhlenhuth was, however, challenged by the void in knowledge which he discovered and spent many subsequent years recording the details from exhaustive anatomical dissections. These works were only partially published before Uhlenhuth's death in 1961. His book is a classic work that should be read and reread by every surgeon who treats neoplastic diseases arising in pelvic structures.

Text continued on page 19.

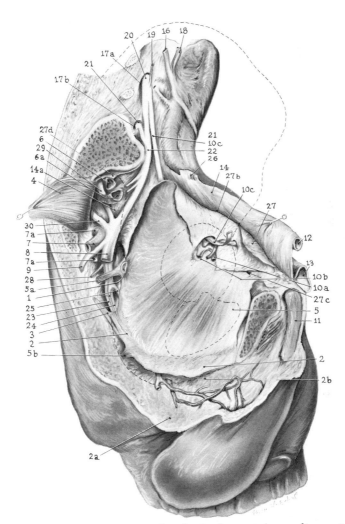

Figure 2–2 1, Ischial spine; 2, pelvic fascia; 3, sacrotuberous ligament; 4, piri-formis muscle; 6, superior gluteal artery; 6a, superior gluteal vein; 7, inferior gluteal artery; 7a, inferior gluteal vein; 8, sciatic nerve; 9, posterior femoral cutaneous nerve; 10a, anterior ramus of obturator artery; 10b, posterior ramus of obturator artery; 10c, obturator nerve; 11, spermatic cord; 12, femoral artery; 13, femoral vein; 14, pectineal ligament; 16, ductus deferens; 17a, fourth lumbar intervertebral foramen; 17b, fifth lumbar foramen; 18, testicular artery and vein; 20, fourth lumbar nerve; 21, fifth lumbar nerve; 22, fourth and fifth lumbar trunks; 23, pudendal nerve; 24, internal pudendal artery; 25, internal pudendal veins. (Anatomic terms for some of the numbered items have been intentionally omitted.)

Figure 2–3 1, Rectum, dorsolateral wall; 2, bladder; 2c, prostate gland; 3, ureter; 4, common iliac artery at the place of bifurcation; 5, kidney; 8, ventral capsule of rectum; 8a, dorsal capsule of rectum; 10, fascia over psoas muscle; 13, presacral wing of visceral fascia; 14, superior wing of visceral fascia; 16, obliterated umbilical artery in preperitoneal (tela subserosa) fascia (vesicoumbilical sheath); 17, preperitoneal fascia in iliac fossa; 17a, preperitoneal fascia on ventral abdominal wall; 18, parietal fascia on iliac muscle; 19, transversalis fascia; 27, pelvic plexus; 28, remnants of parietal fascia left on coccygeus and piriformis muscles; 29, 30, 31 and 32, trunks of sacral nerves S_1, S_2, S_3 and S_4; 33, 34, 35 and 36, sympathetic trunk ganglia 1, 2, 3 and 4, respectively; 37, gangliform body joined by branch from sacral sympathetic ganglion 3 (35); 38, hypogastric nerve (superior hypogastric plexus).

Description: This figure attempts to determine relations of pelvic ganglia. The bladder, rectovesical septum and rectum were reflected forward in order to open up the retrorectal space. The rectum (1) and the presacral wing are now seen from the dorsal view. The dorsal capsule of the rectum (8a) was mobilized; it is seen distinctly that the presacral wing (13) splits along the lateral margin of the rectum into two layers (8a and 8), supplying the ventral and dorsal fascial capsules of the rectum.

It was very easy to raise the dorsal rectal capsule and the presacral wing from the parietal fascia covering the dorsal wall of the pelvis (sacrum, piriformis and coccygeus), but as the rectum was pulled forward, a membranous sheet was stretched which took origin from the parietal fascia in the vicinity of the anterior sacral foramina and passed forward to join the presacral wing and rectal capsule. Enclosed in this sheet were the autonomous nerves as they passed from the sacrum into the presacral wing.

In order to dissect the autonomous nerves, it became necessary to destroy the sheath in which they were enclosed, and in searching for the trunks of the sacral nerves from which the sacral parasympathetic nerves arise, even a large part of the parietal fascia was destroyed (remnants at 28).

Four of the sacral nerve trunks were dissected out and are shown in the illustration (29, 30, 31 and 32); they are S_1, S_2, S_3 and S_4, respectively. Parasympathetic branches were seen arising from S_2 and S_3 (those from S_2 are not shown). The trunk S_3 gave rise to the larger branches; some of these were long, thick nerves which gave rise to several branches each. Most of these branches joined the pelvic plexus, but some of the large nerves arising from S_3 could be followed directly into the dorsal capsule of the rectum where for a considerable distance they passed caudally toward the pelvic floor.

A sympathetic trunk was also dissected out; it was located medial to the sacral foramina and dorsal to the parietal fascia. Four ganglia (33, 34, 35 and 36) were identified, corresponding to the first, second, third and fourth sacral ganglia, respectively. The fourth, or most caudal, ganglion was very small (this illustration, however, does not bear out this statement). The third ganglion (35) was a node of about 1/4" long about 1/8" thick. The second ganglion (34) was small and flat, but the first ganglion (33) was large.

From the third ganglion a large, thick nerve took origin which passed inside the aforementioned fascial sheath into the presacral wing and joined there a flat, gangliform body (37) which received also many parasympathetic branches (not visible). From this gangliform body, a large number of short branches took origin and then passed partly into the rectal capsule and partly into the cranial end of the pelvic plexus.

As the presacral wing was increasingly mobilized, the hypogastric nerve (38), a flat band about 3/16" wide, was seen on its dorsal surface as it passed from cranial to caudal surfaces. It was held to the presacral wing by a thin fascia which was easily removed to free the nerve sufficiently to follow it in its course caudally; it entered the cranial end of the pelvic plexus.

Location of pelvic plexus: The pelvic plexus was enclosed between the two layers of the presacral wing. Its location was determined as follows. Its site corresponded to the junction of the rectovesical septum and presacral wing, just lateral to the fascial capsule of the rectum. As the presacral wing was pulled forward, the plexus was pulled away from the pelvic wall, but in the undisturbed pelvis, it was attached to the pelvic wall just lateral to the rectum. In its craniocaudal extent, it corresponded to a line along which the rectovesical septum is attached to the presacral wing.

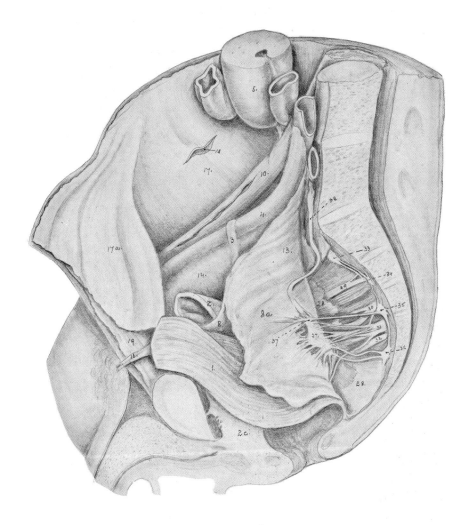

Figure 2–3. *See opposite page for legend.*

Figure 2-4   1, Rectum (muscularis); 2, bladder; 3, ureter; 4, common iliac artery at the point where it branches into external and internal iliac arteries; 5, kidney; 7, rectovesical membrane; 8, capsule of rectum; 9, capsule of bladder; 10, fused parietal and visceral fasciae over psoas muscle, split open; 10a, lateral flap of fascia composed of both psoas fascia and visceral preperitoneal fascia; 10b, psoas (parietal) fascia of medial flap; 10c, visceral preperitoneal fascia of medial flap, continued from superior wing; 10d, deep leaf of iliac sheath was cut away; 11, peritoneum (of rectovesical pouch); 12, peritoneovesical septum; 13, presacral wing of visceral fascia; 14, superior wing of visceral fascia; 15, ductus deferens, horizontal portion; 15a, ductus deferens in retrovesical space; 16, obliterated umbilical artery in visceral preperitoneal fascia; 17, visceral preperitoneal fascia in iliac fossa; 17', visceral preperitoneal fascia on ventral abdominal wall; 18, parietal fascia on iliac muscle; 19, parietal (transverse muscle of abdomen) fascia on ventral abdominal wall.

Description: The peritoneum (11) has been raised by carefully separating it from the fascial leaves; the part of it which lines the rectovesical pouch (11) was preserved and illustrated. The presacral (13) and superior (14) wings of the pelvic fascial sheath are now displayed. The rectovesical membrane (7) is clearly visible; its attachments can be studied. Cranially it is attached to the peritoneum of the rectovesical pouch caudally to the prostate gland; it is a structure distinctly separate from the capsules of the bladder (9) and the rectum (8). The capsule of the rectum (8) proved to be continued cranially.

At 12 a structure is shown which was not found in previous dissections; it is a strong sheet of tissue not unlike, in texture, the peritoneum; it is attached to the peritoneum by its dorsal margin. Ventrally, it is continuous with the capsule of the bladder, whereas laterally it becomes continuous with the superior wing of visceral fascia. In its course, this membrane bridges over the space between bladder and rectovesical septum (the retrovesical space) for which it forms a roof.

The ductus deferens (15) is seen as it lies, in its horizontal course, on top of the superior wing. Along its lateral aspect, it was attached to the superior wing only by loose connective tissue, while along its medial aspect it was attached to this wing by a narrow strip of fascia, a fascial "mesovas." Its dorsal end is seen as it pierces the superior wing at the point where the wing is joined by the fascial membrane (12) to enter the retrovesical space where it is seen at 15a. In the same space, the seminal vesicals are located, but these are not yet visible as they are hidden within the rectovesical membrane.

The superior wing of visceral fascia was followed into the iliac fossa. In the iliac fossa, before any dissection was done, a membrane (17), rather loose in texture but not transparent, could be lifted up with a pair of forceps. It was at first believed that this membrane represented the parietal fascia over the iliac muscle and that, inadvertently, the preperitoneal fascia had been removed when the peritoneum was stripped off. However, when an incision was made into this membrane, the parietal fascia of the iliac muscle (18) was readily displayed, and hence it was proved that the membrane (17) was actually the continuation of the superior wing into the iliac fossa. Ventrally, the continuation of the superior wing (14) into the preperitoneal fascia (17') is shown; it is clearly differentiated from the parietal (or transverse) fascia (19). An incision was then made into the fascia over the psoas muscle (10), and the cut edges were retracted. It was found that in this subject the visceral fascia, as it passed over the psoas, was intimately adherent to the parietal psoas fascia. In the illustration, the lateral cut edge (10a) represents both the visceral and parietal fasciae; after the illustration had been made, a clear-cut separation of these two fasciae along the cut edge was effected. Medially, this separation was made before the illustration was drawn; consequently, the psoas fascia (10b) and the visceral fascia (10c) are seen separately. It was at first not possible to reflect the medial flap of the visceral fascia, since it forms a sheath around the vessels. This sheath was incised; its deep portion (10d) is seen as it dips in between the psoas fascia (10b) and the iliac artery; the cut edge is seen on the superficial portion (10c) of the fascia. Only after this incision had been made and the superficial leaf had been cut away from the deep leaf, the medial flap of the fascia could be reflected and its continuation into the superior wing could be shown.

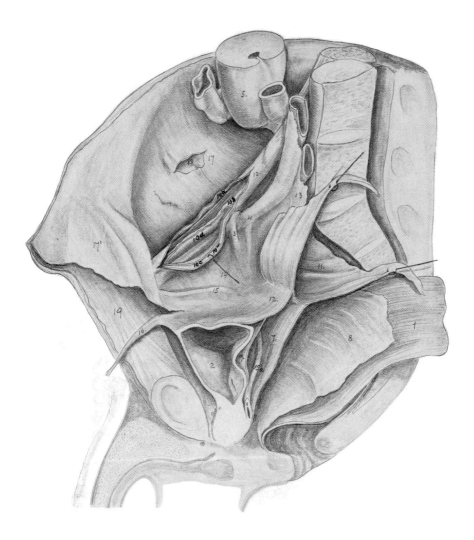

Figure 2–4. *See opposite page for legend.*

Figure 2–5   1, Rectum (muscularis); 2, bladder; 3, ureter; 4, iliac artery at the point of branching into external and internal iliac arteries; 5, kidney; 7, rectovesical septum; 7a, cranial expansion of rectovesical septum into lateral peritoneal wing; 7b, connective tissue bridges between lateral peritoneal wing and rectal capsule (rectal branches of pelvic plexus); 8, capsule of rectum; 9, capsule of bladder; 10, fascia over psoas muscle; 11, peritoneum (rectovesical pouch); 12, peritoneovesical septum; 13, presacral wing of visceral fascia; 14, superior wing of visceral fascia; 15, ductus deferens, horizontal portion; 15a, descending portion of ductus deferens in retrovesical space; 15b, seminal vesicle, dissected free of rectovesical septum (7); 16, obliterated umbilical artery in preperitoneal fascia; 17, preperitoneal fascia in iliac fossa; 17', preperitoneal fascia on ventral abdominal wall; 18, parietal fascia on iliac muscle; 19, parietal (transverse) fascia on ventral abdominal wall.

Description: More work has been done in the retrovesical space. The rectovesical septum (7) has been further separated from the capsule of bladder. The capsule of the seminal vesicle (15b) by which this organ was attached to the ventral surface of the rectovesical membrane has been incised, and the seminal vesical has been separated from the rectovesical membrane. With the finger, spatula and probe the loose connective tissue in the retrovesical space was broken down further laterally, and the lateral attachment of the rectovesical septum was ascertained. It was found that the ductus deferens, in its descending course (15a), is related to the dorsal surface of the inferior pelvic wing of visceral fascia, that the lateral part of the retrovesical space lies between the inferior pelvic wing and the rectovesical septum and that these two fascial membranes are attached laterally along a common line. The beam of a flashlight thrown into the retrovesical space is seen shining through the inferior pelvic wing in the retropubic space.

The capsule of the rectum (8) is seen distinctly continued into the presacral pelvic wing (13); more caudally this wing narrows down, forming specifically a "lateral fascial wing" of the rectum; this is attached laterally to the dorsal surface of the rectovesical septum.

The rectovesical septum shows a cranial expansion into a lateral wing (7a) of the rectovesical pouch of the peritoneum; laterally this lateral wing of the peritoneum is inserted into the presacral wing, close to the lateral margin of the rectal capsule; cranially it ends in a free margin, as shown. On the whole, separation of this lateral peritoneal wing from the presacral wing ventrolaterally and from the rectal capsule dorsomedially is easily accomplished, since the spaces between these membranes are filled only with loose connective tissue. But as the lateral attachment is approached, toughened strands of tissue are encountered, as shown. These are bridges conducting nerves and vessels from the peritoneal wing into the capsule of the rectum. Nearly corresponding to the line of attachment of the peritoneal wing to the presacral wing there lies the pelvic plexus enclosed between the two layers of the presacral wing. This will be shown in Figure 2–3. The tissue bridges (7b) convey the branches of the plexus into the capsule of the rectum.

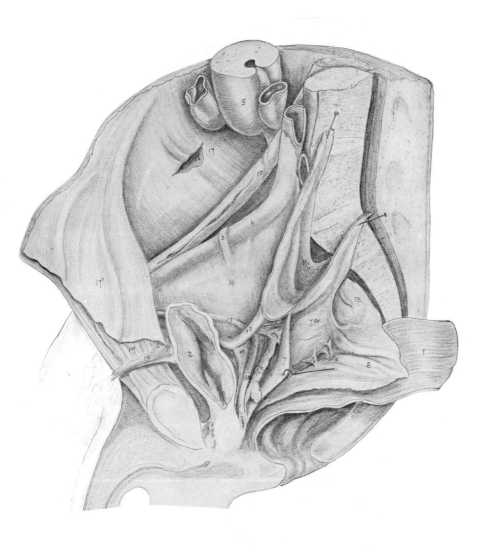

Figure 2–5.   *See opposite page for legend.*

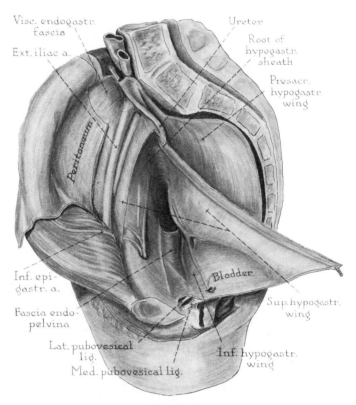

Figure 2–6

When this monograph was started, the authors were already familiar with Uhlenhuth's 1953 work but knew nothing of the man. Consequently, a letter was addressed to Professor Uhlenhuth at the address given in his book. The letter was answered by Professor Frank H. J. Figge, then chairman of the anatomy department and a long-time student of Professor Uhlenhuth. Professor Figge invited one author (J.S.S.) to Baltimore to review Uhlenhuth's extensive files on pelvic anatomy which Uhlenhuth had essentially abandoned after the death of his wife. The original drawings are still preserved in their finest detail and constitute collector's items in themselves. For this text, we reviewed Professor Uhlenhuth's notebooks to select the drawings which we hope will give the working surgeon the clearest perspective of those anatomical relationships that must be understood to perform safe and effective exenterative surgery of the pelvis. A complete presentation of these drawings is unfortunately beyond the scope of this book and is a subject for an anatomical atlas that would update Uhlenhuth's work of 1953 and preserve this wealth of information for many future generations of pelvic surgeons and anatomists. Professor Figge also assumed the task of editing the more recent editions of the *Sobotta-Figge Atlas of Human Anatomy.* This atlas seems to continue Professor Uhlenhuth's example for the use of detailed anatomical studies. All sections of both the Uhlenhuth and Sobotta-Figge atlases covering pelvic anatomy should be studied and learned by the pelvic surgeon with comprehension.

The figures included in this chapter were specifically selected to give the operating surgeon an appreciation of the parietal layer of endopelvic fascia. Between this layer and the musculoskeletal pelvis is the avascular plane in which most dissection must be performed. The authors hold that only surgeons with advanced training and close preceptorial supervision should undertake to perform a pelvic exenteration. The details of anatomy are not as well taught in preceptorial surgical training as are the surgical techniques. Consequently, the anatomy is illustrated in detail and most techniques are described verbally. The written description of the surgical techniques must be read with this anatomical information in mind. The anatomical nomenclature has been updated on all drawings and in the text by Daniel E. Overack, Ph.D., Assistant Professor of Anatomy at the University of Missouri School of Medicine in Columbia, Missouri. The selected illustrations with anatomical legends are contained in Figures 2–1 to 2–17. Ideally, the entire archives of Dr. Uhlenhuth should be published in a single comprehensive edition for the teaching of surgical anatomy.

One additional anatomical illustration is included through the courtesy of Dr. D. B. Slocum. It is Figure 2–18 from *An Atlas of Am-*

Text continued on page 36.

Figure 2-7 1, Symphysis pubis; 2, bladder; 3, rectum; 4, rectovesical pouch; 5, rectovesical septum; 6, cranial continuation of the rectovesical septum; 7, sacrovesical ligament; 8, fascial septum between rectovesical septum and rectal capsule; 9, capsule of rectum; 10, genital fascia; 11, ampulla of ductus deferens and ejaculatory duct; 12, middle lobe of prostate; 13, dorsal lobe of prostate; 14, ureter; 15, superior hypogastric wing of visceral fascia; 16, fascial capsule of superior bladder surface and lateral fascial leaf of inferior pelvic wing; 17, fascial capsule of posterior bladder surface and medial fascial leaf of inferior pelvic wing (margin along which it was cut away from 16); 18, ductus deferens; 19, superior bladder surface; 20, dorsal bladder surface; 21, core of inferior pelvic wing.

Description: The right pelvis of a male seen in a strictly median view. The peritoneum has been stripped away and cut off with the exception of the bottom of the rectovesical pouch (4). Attached to the latter is the rectovesical septum (5). This is prolonged cranially (6) and attached by its lateral margin to the presacral wing of visceral fascia just dorsal to the attachment of the sacrovesical ligament (7). Close to its attachment to the bottom of the pouch, a thin fascial septum (8) connects it to the capsule of the rectum (9). To its ventral surface is attached the genital fascia (10) which splits around the ampulla of the ductus deferens (11) into two layers; the ventral layer is attached to the middle lobe (12), the dorsal layer to the dorsal lobe (13), of the prostate gland.

An incision was made into the fascia of the pelvic root over the ureter (14). The ureter was then shelled out of the fascia to the point where it enters the inferior wing of visceral fascia.

The superior wing (15) was cut through close to the capsule of the bladder; the two edges are seen at 15, 15. This incision was prolonged, dorsally, to the pelvic root, to detach the superior from the inferior wing.

Next, the incision previously made into the pelvic root was prolonged along the inferior wing and further into the capsule of the bladder along the dorsal margin of the superior bladder surface; the cut margins of this incision are seen at 16 and 17. The capsule on the dorsal bladder surface was then peeled away (17); it is continuous with the medial fascial leaf of the inferior wing of visceral fascia. Likewise the capsule on the superior and inferolateral bladder surfaces (16) was peeled away in one continuous layer, together with the lateral fascial leaf of the inferior wing. The unusually high sacrovesical ligament (7), which came along with the dorsomedial fascial leaf, is seen as it passes dorsolaterally to fade away into the presacral wing. The ductus deferens (18), which was cut through when the superior wing (15) was cut through, pierces the fascia and disappears as it enters the retrovesical space.

The inferolateral, superior (19) and dorsal (20) bladder surfaces have thus been freed of the fascial capsule. Likewise the core (21) of the inferior wing has been laid bare; it is seen, in this view, as it attaches itself to the lateral angle of the bladder. Also, its considerable thickness should be noted; where it joins the bladder it is over 1/2 inch thick.

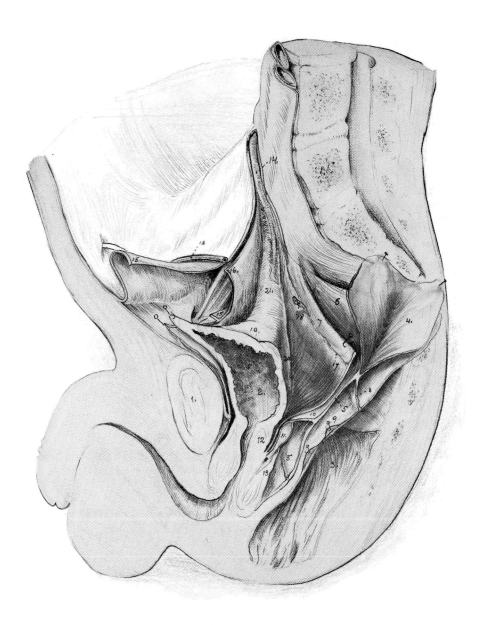

Figure 2–7. *See opposite page for legend.*

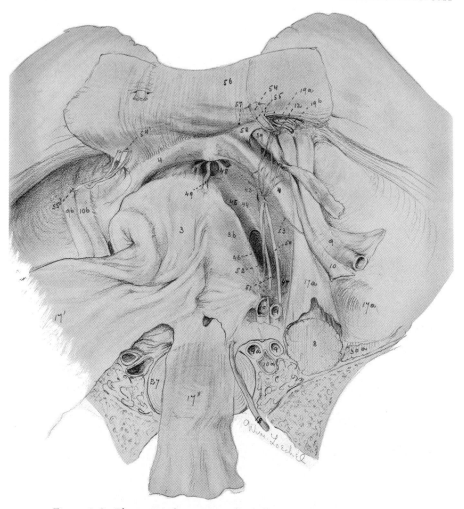

Figure 2–8 The retropubic space. The pelvis has been further cut down to the level of the intervertebral disk between fifth lumbar vertebra and sacrum. The vesico-umbilical fascia and superior wing of visceral fascia have been pulled to the left and dorsally, and the bladder was pulled away from the pelvic walls. 3, Apex of bladder, pulled away from pubic bones and reflected dorsally (covered by fascial capsule); 3b, inferolateral surface of bladder; 4, pectineal crest of superior ramus of pubic bone; 8, psoas (cross section); 9, right external iliac artery; 9a, right internal iliac artery; 9b, left external iliac artery; 10, external iliac vein (right); 10a, right common iliac vein; 10b, left external iliac vein; 12, right ductus deferens (cut off); 17a, muscle fascia (over right psoas and iliac muscles); 17′, preperitoneal fascia (vesicoumbilical fascia); 17″, visceral pelvic fascia (superior wing) plus preperitoneal fascia over iliac fossa, pulled dorsally; 18, right ureter (it is seen dipping into fascia of pelvic root); 19a, right testicular artery; 19b, right testicular vein; 27, intervertebral disk between fifth lumbar vertebra and sacrum; 30a, iliac muscle; 43, obturator fascia; 44, white line of pelvic fascia; 45, lateral ligament of bladder; 46, dorsal continuation of lateral ligament of bladder pelvic fascia, at a deeper level and of more delicate texture; 47, dorsal (vertical) wall of retropubic space (pelvic root) with obturator structures emerging from it; 48, right pubovesical ligament; 49, deep dorsal vein of penis (has not been checked); 50, obturator nerve; 51, obturator artery; 52, obturator vein (to internal iliac system);

Legend continued on opposite page.

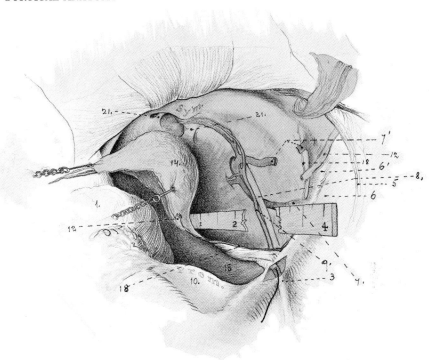

Figure 2-9 Scale 1:1. 1, Sigmoid colon; 3, right ureter, with ureteral catheter in it; 5, internal spermatic vessels; 6, external iliac artery; 6', external iliac vein; 7, obturator vein; 7', anastomosis of obturator vein to external iliac vein; 8, obturator nerve; 9, obturator artery; 10, promontory; 12 and 12, ductus deferens; 14, inferolateral surface of bladder, covered with fascial capsule; 15, presacral wing of visceral fascia; 18 and 18, margins of incision through superior wing of visceral fascia; 21 and 21', right and left medial puboprostatic ligaments. Lateral wall of right retropubic space obturator structures: The right lateral compartment of the retropubic space had been opened up previously by an incision into the superior wing of visceral fascia. The bladder was now pulled over to the left side, and the lateral wall of the right lateral compartment of the retropubic space was illustrated as seen from dorsal and lateral. The depth of the retropubic space was measured; the distance between the floor of the space and the external iliac artery was approximately 3½ inches.

On the lateral wall of the space are seen the obturator structures. The obturator vein had no connection with the internal iliac vein; it opened by two channels (7 and 7') into the external iliac vein. It also received a caudal contribution as well as a ventral contribution which came through the floor of the depression between the left and right puboprostatic ligaments and was evidently the continuation of the deep dorsal veins of the penis. Corresponding branches of the obturator artery were present.

53, obturator vein (to external iliac vein); 54, right inferior epigastric artery (crosses caudal and dorsal to ductus deferens to its origin from external iliac artery); 54', left inferior epigastric artery; 55, tributaries to right inferior epigastric vein; 55', left inferior epigastric vein; 56, transverse fascia; 57, inguinal ligament; 58, lacunar ligament; 59, stout fibroadipose cord containing lymphatics which enter abdominal cavity through femoral ring.

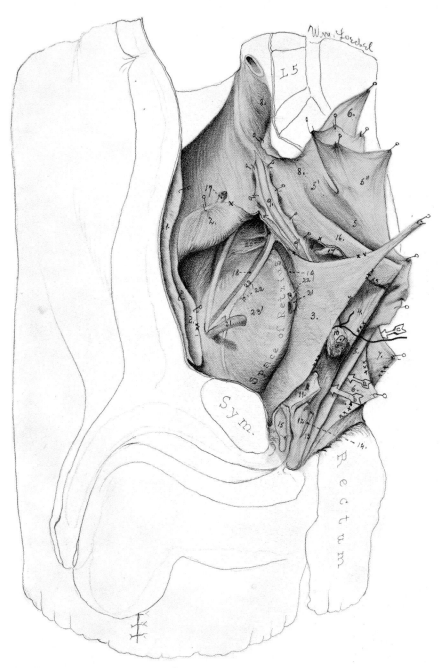

Figure 2–10 1, Preperitoneal on ventral abdominal wall seen from ventromedial; 2 and 2, superior wing of visceral fascia, x margin along which it was cut away from inferior wing, xx margin along which it was cut away from bladder; 3, ventrolateral fascial leaf of inferior wing of visceral fascia, x margin along which it was cut away from superior wing, xx margin along which it was cut away from bladder, xxx median sagittal cut margin; 4 and 4, dorsomedial fascial leaf of inferior wing, x margin along which it was cut away from superior wing, xx margin along which it was cut away from bladder, xxx median sagittal cut margin; 5 and 5, rectovesical septum; 5′, cranial extension of

Legend continued on opposite page.

rectovesical septum; 5″, peritoneum of rectovesical pouch; 6 and 6, ventral fascial capsule of rectum, xxx its median sagittal cut margin; 7, dorsal fascial capsule of rectum, xxx its median sagittal cut margin; 8 and 8, presacral wing of visceral fascia; 9, ureter in pelvic root, at 9′ it enters the inferior wing; 10, vesical cord of inferior wing, with ureter as most cranial structure; 11, trigone which previously had been dissected away from bladder musculature (notice ureteral orifice); 12, middle lobe of prostate, with remnant of bladder wall cranially; 13, dorsal lobe of prostate; 14, ejaculatory duct; 15, ventral lobe of prostate; 16, sacrogenital fold (unusually large); 17 and 17, ductus deferens (cut); 18, obturator vein; 19, inferior vesical vein; 20, common trunk of 18 and 19; 21 and 21, accessory obturator vein (cut) opening into inferior vesical vein 19; 22 and 22, an inferior vesical artery, branching from obturator artery (23); 23′, obturator fascia.

Right half of pelvis, description of dissection composition of inferior wing of visceral fascia and common attachment of five fascial leaves to pelvic fascia: In the previous dissection, the superior wing of visceral fascia had been cut away from the inferior wing; the capsule of the ventrolateral surface of the bladder plus the fascial covering of the ventrolateral surface of the inferior wing had been raised in one continuous fascial sheet and reflected all the way down to the pelvic fascia and pubovesical ligament; the capsule of the dorsal bladder surface and its continuation into the fascial covering of the dorsomedial surface of the inferior wing had been dissected down into the sulcus between middle and posterior lobes of prostate.

Continuation: A more complete display of the various fascial layers was the goal of the following dissection. The dorsal leaf of the inferior wing of visceral fascia was now dissected as far laterally and as far caudally as possible; medially it was lifted out of the prostatic sulcus and then dissected away from the dorsal surface of the posterior lobe all the way down to the prostatic apex; this demonstrated that the dorsal portion of the prostatic capsule is continuous with the dorsomedial leaf of the inferior wing laterally and with the capsule of the bladder cranially.

Next the neurovascular cord of the bladder (vesical cord) was isolated, ligated and cut away from the bladder. The vesical trigone was lifted from the bladder wall, which was cut away, leaving intact the trigonum vesicae and the prostate gland together with the peripheral stump of ureter.

Caudal to the vesical cord another cordlike structure, the prostatic cord, was located, but this is so closely united to the leaves of the inferior wing that isolation would have been possible only by tearing the fascial leaves of the inferior wing. As is indicated in this figure, this cord joins the lateral surface of the lateral lobe of the prostate gland.

Dissection was now started in the retrovesical space, from which the ampulla of the ductus and the seminal vesical had been removed previously. The rectovesical septum was dissected away from the dorsum of the prostate all the way down to the prostatic apex and, laterally, down to its junction with the inferior wing. By means of palpation with the fingers from side of both the retropubic space and the retrovesical space, it was determined that the two fascial leaves of the inferior wing fuse with one another into a single sheet below the prostatic cord.

The prerectal space was then opened up all the way laterally and caudally; this established the fact that the caudal margins of the inferior wing and of the rectovesical septum are fused together into a common attachment to the pelvic fascia.

The retrorectal space was cleaned out, the fascial shelf was displayed, the rectum was shelled out of its capsule and pulled caudally and the dorsal and ventral capsules of rectum were followed into the presacral wing of visceral fascia.

This dissection demonstrates clearly that both leaves of the inferior wing, the rectovesical septum and the presacral wing have a common attachment cranially and dorsally to the pelvic root and caudally and ventrally to the pelvic fascia. The common attachment to the pelvic fascia is mediated by the inferior wing, since both the rectovesical septum and presacral wing in this case fused with the inferior wing somewhat cranial to its attachment to the pelvic fascia. If the fingers of one hand are introduced into the retropubic space and the other hand is placed into the retrorectal space, the common fascial sheet of attachment can be distinctly verified. Moreover, if the five fascial wings are grasped and pulled in the direction away from their attachment, the beam of a flashlight thrown into the retropubic space is seen through the common sheet of attachment in the retrorectal space.

A wire frame was built and placed over the specimen. Strings with hooks were attached to each one of the five fascial leaves; these were stretched, and the strings were fastened to the frame. In this way the fascial leaves could be spread out and their mutual relations distinctly seen.

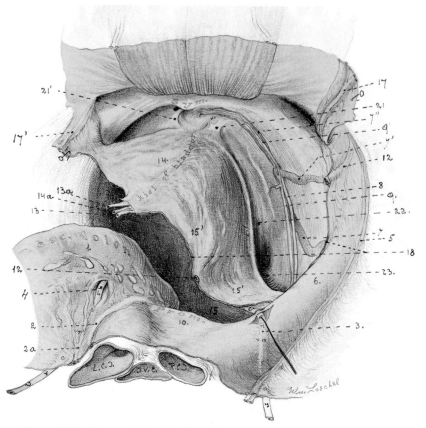

Figure 2–11 Floor and dorsal wall of the retropubic space. 1, Sigmoid colon; 2, superior rectal artery; 2a, sigmoid artery; 3, right ureter with ureteral catheter in it; 4, left ureter, crossing external iliac artery under root of sigmoid mesocolon; 5, right internal spermatic vessels; 6, external iliac artery; 7, obturator vein; 7′, anastomosis of obturator vein to external iliac vein; 7″, tributary of obturator vein coming through floor of depression between medial puboprostatic ligaments; 8, obturator nerve; 9, obturator artery; 9′, branch of obturator artery, perforating floor of depression between medial pubovesical ligaments; 10, promontory; 12 and 12, ductus deferens, cut through and reflected with superior wing of visceral fascia (15′); 13 and 13a, right and left umbilical arteries; 14, left ventrolateral surface of bladder; 14a, urachus; 15, presacral wing of visceral fascia; 15′ and 15′, superior wing of visceral fascia; 17 and 17′, inferior epigastric vessels; 18, margins of incision into superior wing of visceral fascia; 21 and 21′, right and left medial puboprostatic ligaments; 22, floor of retropubic space (pelvic fascia); 23, dorsal wall of retropubic space (pelvic root), greatly foreshortened; I.V.C., inferior vena cava; L.C.I. and R.C.I., left and right common iliac arteries.

Floor and dorsal wall of the retropubic space: The superior wing of visceral fascia and the bladder are now fully pulled to the left, and the right lateral compartment of the retropubic space is illustrated from above so that both its floor and its dorsal wall can be seen; the dorsal wall, however, is greatly foreshortened.

On the right side the medial puboprostatic ligament stands out prominently. It is followed dorsally by the pelvic fascia (22). At 23 the pelvic root still covered with fascia is seen.

The depression between the two puboprostatic ligaments is illustrated; the vessels perforating its floor, an artery and two veins do not anastomose with the vesical plexus but are branches of the obturator vessels.

On the left side the ureter (4) was dissected out where it crossed the iliac artery under the root of the sigmoid mesocolon.

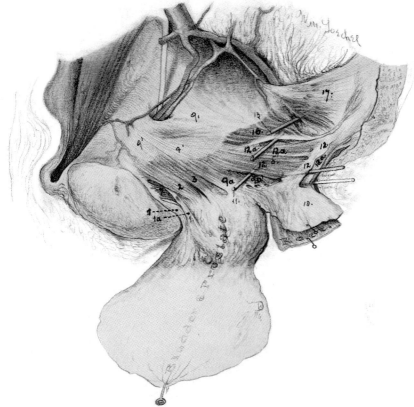

Figure 2–12 1, 2, 3, 4, 5 and 5′, Pubococcygeus; 1, pubococcygeus inserted into ventral aspect of prostatic capsule (possibly puboprostatic ligament); 2 and 3, pubococcygeus bundles inserted into lateral prostatic capsule; 4, pubococcygeus bundle inserted into dorsal prostatic and ventral rectum capsule; 5, pubococcygeus inserted into rectum; 5′, pubococcygeus inserted into general levator aponeurosis; 6, iliococcygeus; 7, coccygeus; 8, general levator aponeurosis of insertion; 8′, probably anococcygeal raphe of iliococcygeus; 9, obturator fascia; 9′, tendon of origin of pubococcygeus from pubic bone; 10, rectal capsule; 11, 12 and 13, probes separating individual portions of levator.

Description: The rectum was cut through and both ends reflected, but only the caudal end, still covered with its fascial capsule (10), is shown in the drawing. All visceral fasciae are cut away from the line of anchorage and reflected upward; they are not shown. The parietal fascia is then carefully removed from the pelvic floor muscles as far cranially as the ischial spine and superior margin of coccygeus (7).

The arcus tendineus is not distinct here; at present the line of origin of the levator cannot be determined with accuracy except the origin directly from the pubic bone. Pubococcygeus and iliococcygeus are well defined; the boundary between them is marked by the probe no. 12.

The pubococcygeus presents so far six separate portions. The most ventral portion (1) consists of narrow fiber bundles arising close to the lower end of the symphysis pubis; it passes to the prostate and fades out on the fascial capsule of it. The next two groups of bundles (2 and 3) are both inserted into the lateral aspect of the prostatic capsule. The fourth group (4′) is inserted partly into the dorsal aspect of prostatic capsule (9a) and partly into the ventral capsule of the rectum (9a). The fifth group (9a′) is inserted into the rectal capsule by means of connective tissue cords. The sixth group (12), which seems to lie at a more cranial level, is inserted into the sacrum by means of the aponeurosis of insertion (12). Below this lies a sheet of tissue (12a) which is probably part of the iliococcygeus and might represent the anococcygeal raphe. The part of the iliococcygeus visible so far (16) is of small size; from its origin it tapers down to a tendinous narrow band which seems to be inserted into the general aponeurosis of insertion (12). The coccygeus (17) is inserted into the bone of sacrum and coccyx.

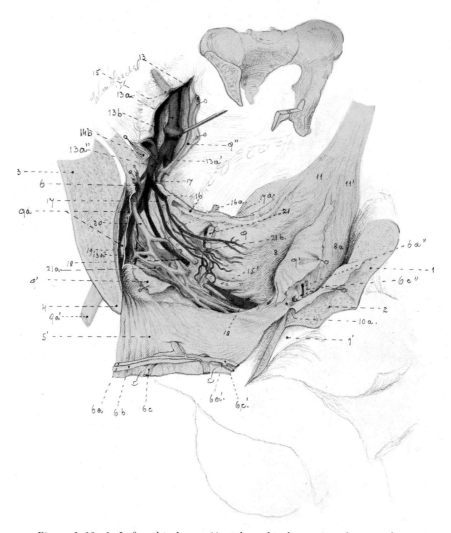

Figure 2–13 1, Left pubic bone; 1', right pubic bone; 2, pubic symphysis; 3, ilium; 4, ischial spine; 5', internal obturator fascia; 6, central stump of obturator artery with obturator nerve; 6a, 6b and 6c, peripheral stumps of obturator artery, nerve and vein; 6a' and 6c', ventral branches of obturator artery and vein; 6a" and 6c", peripheral stumps of branches of obturator artery and vein, entering retropubic fossa; 8 and 8a, right and left ventrolateral bladder surfaces covered with fascial capsule; 9, ventral wing of visceral fascia; 9', flaps of lateral fascial leaf peeled off the ventral wing to expose nerves and vessels; 9", flap of ventral fascial leaf of pelvic root (transition from presacral wing into ventral hypogastric wing); 10a, right puboprostatic ligament; 11 and 11', right and left vesicoumbilical fascia; 13, common iliac artery; 13a, internal iliac artery; 13b, external iliac artery; 13a., posterior division of internal iliac artery; 13a" and 13a", anterior division of internal iliac artery; 14b, external iliac vein; 15, ureter crossing iliac artery; 15', ureter in inferior wing, transected to expose ductus deferens and genital artery; 16, umbilical artery, transected; 16a, superior vesical artery; cranial branch to superior bladder surface, caudal branch to lateral bladder surface and ureter; 17, vesicogenital artery; cranial branch to bladder caudal branch gives off deferential artery to ductus deferens (21), a ventral branch to ureter and a caudal or genital branch which perforates the medial fascial leaf of inferior wing and passes into retrovesical space; 18 and 18, vesicoprostatic artery, transected; 19, prostatic artery; 20, internal iliac vein; 21a and 21b, two ganglionic masses (parts of pelvic plexus) which were con-

Legend continued on opposite page.

nected by an anastomosis; this was lateral to the ureter and was cut through. The cranial ganglion sends branches to the bladder, the caudal ganglion mostly to prostate; 21, ductus deferens.

Contents of inferior wing: obturator artery (6) – only the central stump has been left attached to the internal iliac artery; the rest (6a) is on the reflected flap (5'). The umbilical artery (16) is the most cranial artery in the superior wing. Shortly after its origin, it gives rise to a superior vesical (16a). This breaks up into two branches; the cranial branch is distributed to the superior bladder surface, while the caudal branch supplies the lateral bladder surface. The vesicoprostatic artery (18) is a very large and long vessel, as can be seen. It lies in its entirety in the inferior wing, runs approximately parallel (and caudal) to the ureter and forms part of the vesical cord. It gives off several branches to the lateral bladder surface, passes forward and disappears under the pubovesical ligament on the lateral surface of the prostate gland. For a short distance the vesicogenital artery (17) passes in caudal direction within the pelvic root, enters the superior wing and passes forward and disappears under the pubovesical ligament on the lateral surface of the prostate gland. It then breaks up into two branches. The smaller cranial branch enters the capsule on the lateral bladder surface; the larger caudal branch represents the genital artery. In its peripheral course it is remarkable by its tortuousness. It gives off an artery to the ductus deferens which is closely attached to the dorsal surface of the ductus deferens and appears more like the continuation of the main vessel than a branch of it. After giving rise to the artery to the ductus deferens artery, its diameter is notably decreased; it passes caudally and pierces the medial leaf of the inferior wing to enter the retrovesical space.

The main vessel and its caudal genital branch take about the same course as the ureter. At first the vessel is lateral to the ureter, but it finally crosses over the ventro-cranial aspect of the ureter and descends on the medial side of the ureter. The prostatic artery (19) takes a long caudal course in which it crosses medial to the sacral parasympathetic nerves and is located in the pelvic root. At the caudal end of this course, the artery lies below the floor of the retropubic space. It then turns abruptly forward, remaining for the rest of its course below the pelvic fascia; the horizontal course is about the same length as the vertical course. In its horizontal course, it divides into two stout branches which enter the lateral surface of the prostate gland. In this subject, the vertical part of the artery was much thinner than the horizontal part. Both the vesical and the prostatic venous plexuses were abundantly developed and dissected, but only a part of the prostatic plexus was illustrated. The entire plexus collects into a single vein (20), an internal iliac vein. On the whole, the veins form the most superficial stratum. Measured from the side of the retropubic space, along the ductus, the ureter lies 38 mm. caudal to the umbilical artery. Of the visceral nerves, only two ganglionic masses (21a and 21b) are visible; the two were connected by an anastomotic branch which, however, was divided in order to expose the ureter and genital artery. One ganglionic mass (21b) supplies the ureter and bladder, the other (21a) supplies the prostate. Localization of ureter: to find the ureter in the inferior lying wing from the caudal side (i.e., from the side of the space of Retzius) the distance of the ureter from the obliterated umbilical artery, measured along the ductus deferens, is 38 mm. (about 7½ inches).

Contents of inferior wing: the pelvic fascia is separated from its attachments to inferior wing and presacral wing of visceral fascia. The lateral fascial leaf of the ventral wing has been dissected away to expose the contents of the ventral wing; parts, however, are still present and have been illustrated (9, 9' and 9"). Dorsally the lateral leaf becomes continuous with the dorsal wall of the retropubic space. Since the attachments of inferior wing and presacral wing have been cut away from the pelvic fascia, the two wings appear now in continuity with one another along the margin of their common attachment. In this figure, however, the dissection is confined to the inferior wing.

The medial fascial leaf has been left entirely intact. It forms, as can be seen, the medial wall of the pelvic root and becomes continuous with the ventral leaf of the presacral wing. The first two arteries arising from the anterior division of the internal iliac artery are the vesicogenital (17) and the obturator (6); they arise just opposite each other. The umbilical (16) and the vesicoprostatic (18) arteries arise by a common trunk, somewhat caudal to the foregoing arteries. The last artery arises separately, caudal to the common trunk of 16 and 18; it is the prostatic artery (19), a vessel of considerable size.

Figure 2-14   1, Symphysis pubis; 2, fifth lumbar vertebra; 3_{1-5}, sacral vertebrae; 4, coccyx; 5, superior pubic ramus; 5a, inferior pubic ramus; 6, piriformis muscle; 7, internal obturator; 8, unidentified muscle (probably aberrant bundle of obturator internus inserted into rectal fascia); 9, coccygeal muscle, tendinous part (with sharp crescentic margin); 9a and 9b, coccygeal muscle, fleshy bundles inserted into coccyx; 9c, coccygeal muscle, fleshy bundle inserted into fascia over sphincter ani; 10a, levator ani, lateral flap created by dividing the muscle; 10b and 10c, levator ani (and fascia), medial flap; 10b, superficial layer, 10c, deep layer, 10d, deep transverse perineal; 11, sacrococcygeal (ventral): lateral bundle arises from tendon of coccygeus muscle, medial bundle from periosteum on sacrum; 12, remnant of parietal fascia over piriformis and coccygeus; 13, remnant of internal obturator fascia; 14, part of obturator fascia forming pudendal neurovascular bundle was exposed; 15, probably fused superior urogenital and inferior levator fasciae; 16, cut margin of parietal fascia which clips in between internal obturator and coccygeus; 17, presacral root; 18, common iliac artery; 19, external iliac artery; 20, external iliac vein; 21, superior gluteal artery; 22, inferior lateral sacral artery; 23, superior lateral sacral artery; 24, one inferior gluteal vein; 25a, 25b and 25c, first, second and third sacral nerves (anterior divisions); 26, ischiorectal fossa; 27, obturator artery; 28, obturator nerve; 29, obturator vein; 30, anastomosis between inferior gluteal artery and internal pudendal artery; 31, anastomosis between venous plexus just proximal to branching into three veins — internal pudendal and two inferior gluteal veins; 32a, internal pudendal vein (at the point at which it disappears dorsal to the coccygeal muscle); 33a, internal pudendal artery (at the point at which it disappears dorsal to the coccygeal muscle); 32a and 33b, same vessels after emergence from coccygeal muscle into perineum. The location of the ischial spine and ischial tuberosity are marked by black dots.

Levator ani: the medial flap is probably the part of the caudal surface which formed the medial boundary of the ischiorectal fossa (26); it contained two distinct layers (10b and 10c). The nature of the muscle 10d is not quite clear; it may be the deep transverse perineal muscle or a part of levator ani. Obturator fascia: the fascia (14) is that part of the perineal obturator fascia which contained the internal pudendal neurovascular bundle. The fascia labeled 15, although continuous with 14, is considerably thicker and tougher and seems to consist of several layers; it is probably the product of fusion of superior urogenital with inferior levator fascia. Pudendal vessels: the branching of anterior division of internal iliac artery into inferior gluteal and internal pudendal arteries occurred in the pelvic cavity within the hypogastric root, 50 mm. proximal to the superior margin of the coccygeus muscle; the arterial perineopelvic anastomosis therefore existed between the pelvic and perineal portions of the same artery (internal pudendal).

The internal iliac vein formed from three branches, a superior (24) and an inferior (not visible) "inferior gluteal" veins and a pudendal vein; where these three veins met, a stout venous plexus was formed which gave rise to the internal iliac vein. The venous perineopelvic anastomosis joined the pudendal vein just proximal to the point where the pudendal vein joined the plexus; the distal end of this anastomosis joined the pudendal vein just distal to the inferior margin of the coccygeal muscle.

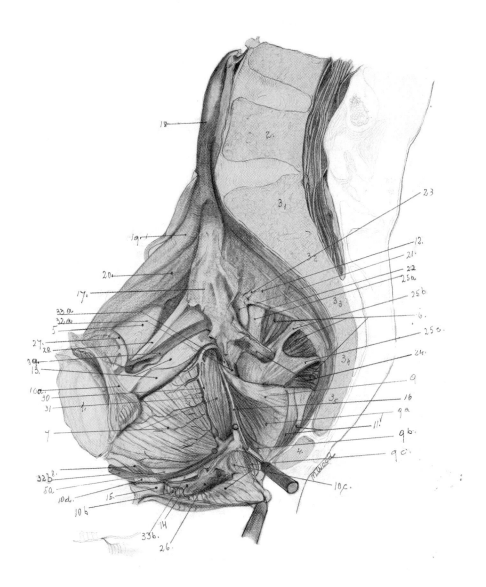

Figure 2–14. *See opposite page for legend.*

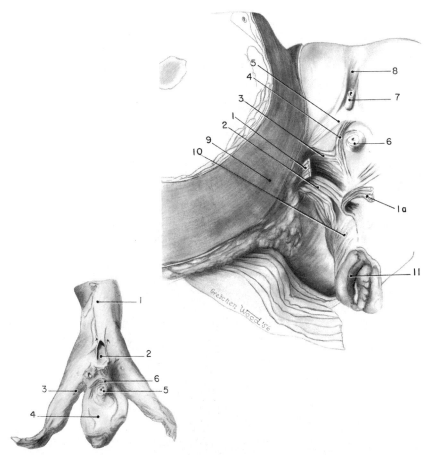

Figure 2-15 Left, 1, Corpus cavernosum penis; 2, vein of penis; 3, crus (left) corpus cavernosum; 4, bulb of corpus spongiosum; 5, membranous urethra; 6, sphincter urethrae muscle. *Right,* 1, levator ani (pubococcygeus); la, levator ani (pubococcygeus); 2, levator ani (iliococcygeus); 3, pubococcygeus (puborectalis); 4, pubococcygeus (levator prostatae); 5, arcuate ligament; 6, prostate; 7, dorsal vein of penis; 8, pubic symphysis; 9, fascia lata femoris; 10, rectum (external and sphincter); 11, anus.

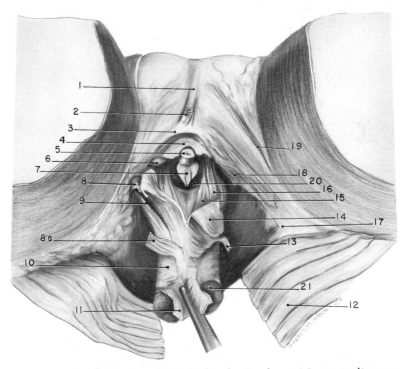

Figure 2-16 1, Pubic symphysis; 2, dorsal vein of penis; 3, arcuate ligament; 4, puboprostatic ligament; 5, urethra; 6, arcus tendineus; 7, prostate; 8, inferior recto-urethralis; 8a, inferior rectourethralis; 9, superior rectourethralis; 10, rectum (external anal sphincter); 11, central point of perineum; 12, iliococcygeus muscle; 14, pubo-coccygeus; 15, pubococcygeus (levator prostatae); 16, pubococcygeus (puborectalis); 17, ischial tuberosity; 18, fascia of urogenital diaphragm; 19, ischiopubic ramus.

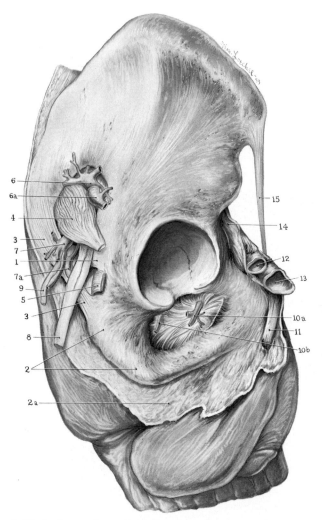

Figure 2-17 1, Sacrospinous ligament; 2, superior ramus of ischium; 3, sacro-tuberous ligament; 4, piriformis muscle; 5, internal obturator muscle; 6, superior gluteal artery; 6a, superior gluteal vein; 7, inferior gluteal artery; 7a, inferior gluteal vein; 8, sciatic nerve; 9, posterior femoral cutaneous nerve; 10a, anterior ramus of obturator artery; 10b, posterior ramus of obturator artery; 11, spermatic cord; 12, femoral artery; 13, femoral vein; 14, pectineal ligament; 15, inguinal ligament.

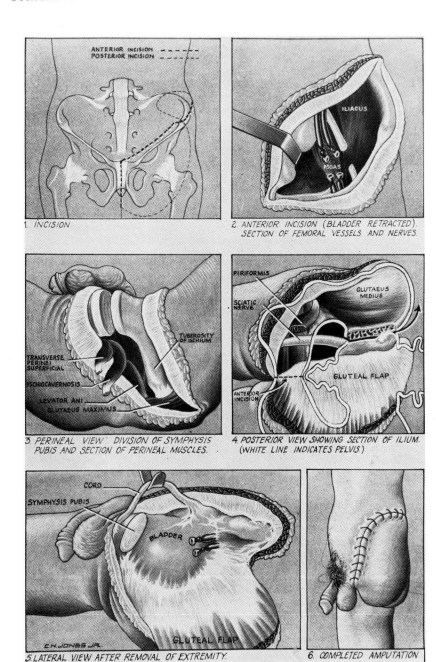

Figure 2-18 Hindquarter amputation (technique of King and Steelquist). (Reprinted from Slocum, Donald B.: An Atlas of Amputations. St. Louis, the C. V. Mosby Co., 1949.)

putations, published by The C. V. Mosby Company in 1949. The illustration gives a clear view of pelvic anatomy requisite to perform a hemipelvectomy when this is occasionally required en bloc with an exenteration of the pelvic viscera.

REFERENCES

Figge, F. H. J.: Eduard Uhlenhuth, 1885–1961. Anat. Rec., *143*:278, 1962.
Figge, F. H. J.: Personal communication, 1971.
Slocum, D. B.: An Atlas of Amputations. St. Louis, The C. V. Mosby Co., 1949.
Sobotta, J.: Atlas of Human Anatomy. 8th ed. Vols. 1–3. Revised by F. H. J. Figge. New York, Hafner Publishing Company, Inc., 1963.
Uhlenhuth, E.: Problems in the Anatomy of the Pelvis, An Atlas. Philadelphia, J. B. Lippincott Co., 1953.

Chapter Three

INDICATIONS,
CONTRAINDICATIONS
AND END RESULTS

Every patient with a biopsy-proven neoplasm in a pelvic viscus that is either not curable by a lesser operation or that has recurred in the pelvis after an adequate dose of radiation therapy or after a lesser surgical procedure should be considered as a potential candidate for a pelvic exenteration. Proven metastases outside the confines of the true pelvis are categorical contraindications. Other variables are of great significance in the selection of candidates for surgery.

In general, every patient with the above circumstances who is mentally competent and possesses a will to live, who does not have a serious medical problem that would make prolonged anesthesia and the administration of banked blood intolerable, who does not have another incurable problem associated with a life expectancy of at least 24 months and who can provide an informed consent for the procedure is a candidate.

The fact that pelvic exenteration can be curative for many advanced pelvic cancers is attributable to intrinsic biological characteristics of many of these cancers. The significant characteristic is that they can grow to great size, involving adjacent organs by contiguous invasion, and yet not metastasize. They are chronic local cancers which are capable of producing extensive local destruction, urinary and enteric obstruction, hemorrhage secondary to the dissolution of major blood vessels, intractable pain from neural invasion, inanition, sepsis and death of the host. The death is the end result of progressive

37

local growth and its side effects. This chronic local variant of cancer probably comprises between 20 and 60 per cent of all pelvic cancers—more for some morphological variants and less for others. Some cancers that do metastasize to lymph nodes may have their metastases restricted to a very few lymph nodes in close proximity to the primary cancer. These may still be controlled by exenterative surgery. When more than several lymph nodes in the pelvis or any lymph nodes outside the pelvis along the aorta contain metastases surgical cure is unreported.

An understanding of the dynamics of tumor growth and host response to the cancer's presence affords some appreciation of why

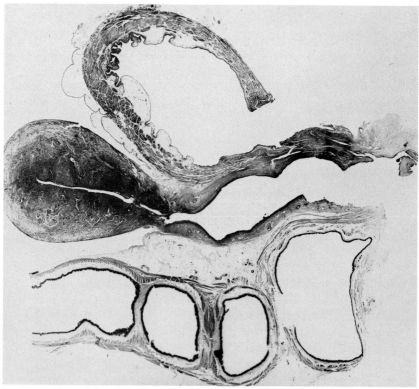

Figure 3–1   (70-39238) This woman was first admitted to the radiotherapy service in 1970 with a stage III epidermoid carcinoma of the cervix uteri which was treated by radiotherapy. By late 1970 it had recurred, and a total pelvic exenteration was performed, producing the specimen shown here. The pathologist described it as a post-irradiationally persistent and degenerating epidermoid carcinoma. Extensive chronic inflammation and fat necrosis were present in the pelvic soft tissues, including bullous edema of the bladder. The cancer was not controlled, however, and she developed generalized carcinomatosis and died. Currently, this patient would have a scalene lymph node biopsy to exclude the presence of metastases before receiving any form of radical treatment. (Courtesy of Dr. Carlos Perez-Mesa.)

these pelvic cancers can become so extensive before being detected and still remain localized. The in vivo growth rate of cancers growing in the pelvic organs of man has not been measured. The pulmonary metastases from them grow with median (log mean) doubling times of 65 days with a range of 2 standard deviations (95 per cent) from 8 to 512 days (Spratt, 1964). If the cancer is a surface growing neoplasm with continual desquamation, the net growth rate is much slower. Comparatively, the median doubling time of primary colorectal adenocarcinomas is 620 days, but the median doubling time from pulmonary metastases from this group of cancers is 109 days. The number of net doublings required for one cancer cell to produce a mass of neoplasm large enough to diagnose is between 20 and 30. However, most neoplasms will have killed the host before the fortieth doubling. Also, the Weber-Fechner law physiologically determines the inclina-

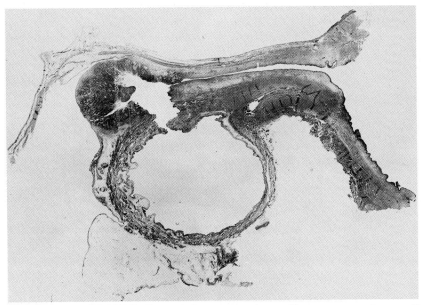

Figure 3–2   (68-37694) This specimen comes from a Negro woman who was 48 years old when first seen at the EFSCH in 1968. In 1967 she had a hysterectomy at another institution followed by a one-month course of external radiotherapy. The pathological slides obtained from the other hospital were read as showing mid-differentiated epidermoid carcinoma of the cervix uteri with extensive infiltration of the cervix and questionable extension into paracervical soft tissue. She was referred to EFSCH after she developed recurrent vaginal bleeding. Because of the localized nature of the recurrence, it was treated with radium in February, 1969; by September of that year the cancer was again palpable in the upper vagina with probable bladder invasion and possible vesicovaginal fistula. On 9-30-69, a pelvic exenteration was performed. Preoperative biopsies were read as showing poorly differentiated cancer. The cancer in the exenteration specimen was read as showing predominantly mid-differentiated cancer. Only 1 of 20 lymph nodes contained metastatic cancer. She remained free of recurrent cancer and was gaining weight when seen on last follow-up in the clinic in 1972. (Courtesy of Dr. Carlos Perez-Mesa.)

tion of hosts stimulated by the symptoms from these neoplasms to seek medical aid. This law states that man's response to stimuli (i.e., cancer size) varies according to a log normal distribution of the magnitude of this stimulus. Whether sensitivity can be increased by patient education is unknown, but the success of such an effort for visceral cancers would be doubtful. Thus, in the absence of actual early detection by physical or laboratory examination performed frequently enough to avoid the growth of large cancers, a respectable percentage of patients with pelvic neoplasms will always have very large cancers. By multiplying the doubling times by the 10 or 20 doublings elapsing between the growth of a cancer large enough to diagnosis and one large enough to kill, it can be seen that the time range between susceptibility to diagnosis and lethality may range from a few months to many years. This time range will be lognormally distributed as will the size of cancers actually diagnosed (Spratt, 1969). The variance of size range of adenocarcinomas of the colon and rectum at the time of diagnosis is from 2.8 to 13.2 cm. with a median of 6.1 cm. if the cancers have a biological propensity to metastasize to lymph nodes and from 2.8 to 13.7 cm. with a median of 6.2 cm. if the cancers are not inclined

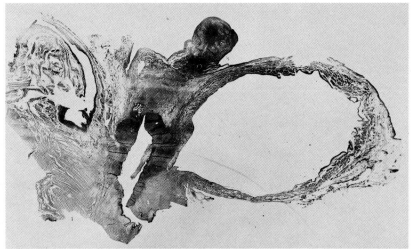

Figure 3–3 (69-38383) The woman from whom this specimen was taken was first seen at the EFSCH at the age of 63. Thirteen years before, she had received radiotherapy for carcinoma of the cervix uteri (stage unknown) at another institution. The recurrent cancer was read as being highly undifferentiated with a spindle cell pattern. The possibility that the neoplasm was a leiomyosarcoma could not be excluded. The cancer had grown by direct extension into the paracervical tissues, the urinary bladder and the vagina, as confirmed on examination of the specimen obtained from the exenteration on 8-26-69. This cancer was not a biologically favorable variant for control by any form of ablative surgery. She had a transient period of palliation and died of a massive local recurrence and generalized metastases on 4-12-71. (Courtesy of Dr. Carlos Perez-Mesa.)

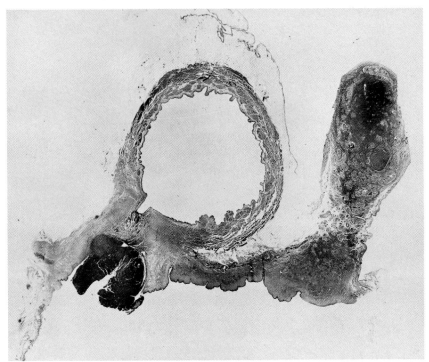

Figure 3–4   (67-36097) This specimen comes from an anterior pelvic exenteration performed on 2-5-67 for a mid-differentiated epidermoid carcinoma of the urethra. Lymph nodes in the pelvic exenteration specimen contained no metastases. However, inguinal lymph nodes became palpable, and a bilateral groin dissection was performed on 3-26-68. One of nine nodes from the left groin and one of twelve nodes from the right contained metastatic cancer. She expired on 4-30-69 of generalized skeletal metastases. At the time of death she also was developing nodules in the pubic skin. The biological behavior of this urethral cancer was not favorable for control by pelvic exenteration, although this could not have been predicted at the time of surgery. Even now the total experience with urethral cancer remains limited. (Courtesy of Dr. Carlos Perez-Mesa.)

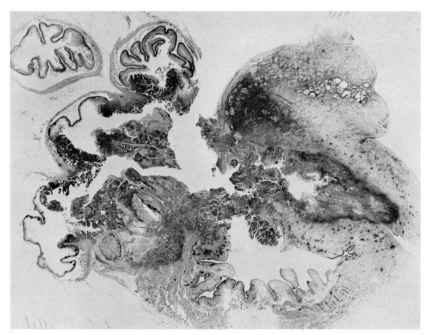

Figure 3–5   (63-32077) The woman from whom this specimen was taken first had a sigmoidectomy in 1963 for mid-differentiated adenocarcinoma extending through the colonic wall with perforation and abscess formation. Three of 12 lymph nodes contained metastatic cancer. For extensive pelvic recurrence with multiple enteroenteric and uterovesical fistulas, an anterior pelvic exenteration was performed in 1966, producing the specimen in this figure. She died in 1969 with generalized adenocarcinomatosis. In addition to the biological propensity to remain and recur locally for a long period of time, it is quite possible that the growth rate of this neoplasm was quite slow. (Giant section courtesy of Dr. Carlos Perez-Mesa.)

to metastasize. There is no significant difference between the size distributions of this to biological variants (Spratt, 1970). Thus, the data for colon cancer particularly well document how large the cancers can become without metastasis.

Gross photographs and giant histological sections of pelvic exenteration specimens (courtesy of Dr. Carlos Perez-Mesa) have been selected to demonstrate the extraorgan extension and multiple organ involvement of various pelvic cancers (Figs. 3–1 to 3–8). These figures all demonstrate transgression by cancer of the visceral layer of fascia around the organ in which the cancer originates. When this occurs, the next plane for avascular dissection circumscribing the neoplasm is usually between the parietal layer of endopelvic fascia and the musculoskeletal pelvis, thus requiring a pelvic exenteration.

The actual experience with the performance of pelvic exenteration is considered by anatomical site. At the completion of the discussion by sites, a summary table of end results is given. The actuarial method used in calculating the end results is given in Appendix 1.

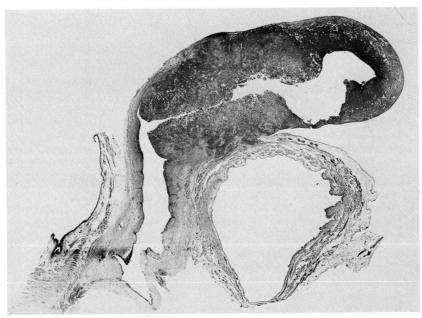

Figure 3–6   (65-34408) This woman received telecobalt and intracavitary curietherapy for a stage IIa mid-differentiated epidermoid carcinoma of the cervix uteri in 1965. On 9-6-66 she underwent a total pelvic exenteration for postirradiationally recurrent cancer. Histological examination showed the cancer had extended to the body of the uterus, vagina, pericervical soft tissue and wall of the urinary bladder. None of 15 lymph nodes present in the exenteration specimen contained metastatic cancer. (Giant section courtesy of Dr. Carlos Perez-Mesa.)

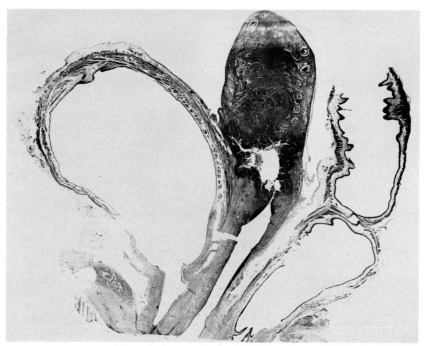

Figure 3–7   (66-35614) This giant section comes from the total pelvic exenteration specimen of a 53-year-old woman. She had received radiotherapy at another institution for a stage I carcinoma of the cervix uteri and was referred to the EFSCH because of recurrent carcinoma. On admission examination the vagina was atrophic and admitted only one finger. The entire circumference of the cervix was necrotic, and this necrosis extended into the upper third of the vagina on the left side. On rectal examination the paracervical tissue on the left was hard and thickened. The intravenous pyelogram showed no ureteropathy. On 8-16-66 the patient underwent a total exenteration.

Histological examination of the resected specimen confirmed postirradiationally persistent mid-differentiated squamous cell cancer with direct extension into the body of the uterus and urinary bladder. The vagina contained extensive carcinoma in situ. None of the lymph nodes in the removed specimen contained metastatic cancer. (Giant section courtesy of Dr. Carlos Perez-Mesa.)

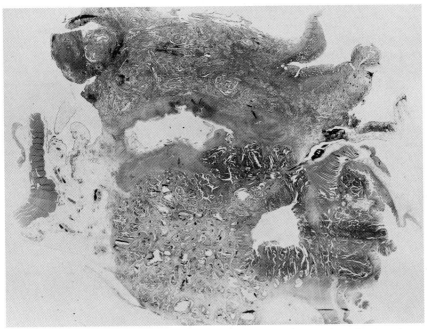

Figure 3–8 (67-36280) This giant section demonstrates a mucin-producing adeno-carcinoma of the rectum that measured 9 cm. in its greatest chordal dimension. The cancer extended through the bowel wall into the pericolonic fat. None of 20 lymph nodes contained metastases in spite of the size and extent of the cancer. The specimen was removed by posterior exenteration from a 74-year-old woman. (Giant section courtesy of Dr. Carlos Perez-Mesa.)

ANUS

Anal cancer has been an indication for exenterative pelvic surgery in only three cases at the EFSCH and Barnes Hospital (Table 3–1). Posterior exenteration has been universally associated with a non-functioning bladder. The bladder is completely denervated by the lateral and posterior dissection, and an ileal bladder is less trouble to manage. As a result, exenterations performed for anal or rectal cancers should be total. Adequate surgery for anal cancers does require wide excision of the perianal skin along with abdominoperineal resection in most cases (Dillard). Inguinal nodes are resected by groin dissection when they are involved. However, involvement of other pelvic viscera is infrequent. There is rarely an indication for simultaneous pelvic exenteration and groin dissections in these cases. When possible, the operations should be staged. If there is any question about involvement of the superficial inguinal lymph nodes, the lymphatic bundle passing through the inguinopectineal triangle must be ligated at the time of the exenterative resection of the anorectum (Spratt,

Table 3–1   End Results at Barnes Hospital and EFSCH

	NUMBER OF EXENTERA- TIONS	DEATHS WITHIN 30 DAYS OF EXENTERA- TION	HOSPITAL MORTALITY RATE (per cent)	ACCUMULATIVE SURVIVAL RATES* (per cent)		
				1 yr.	*3 yr.*	*5 yr.*
Cervix						
EFSCH						
Anterior	10	1	10	80	70	56
Modified	3	0	0	33	0	0
Total exenterations	52	5	9	61	47	47
All cases	65	6	9	61	48	42
Barnes Hospital						
All cases	209	17	8	78	51	39
Rectum and sigmoid						
EFSCH	21	2	9	49	21	21
Barnes Hospital	43	7	16	75	60	45
Corpus uteri						
EFSCH						
Anterior	8	1	13	58	29	29
Total	6	1	17	33	22	22
Bladder						
EFSCH	50	6	12	64.6	44.7	37.85
Barnes Hospital	4	0	0	25	0	0
Urethra						
EFSCH	2	2	100	0	0	0
Barnes Hospital	2	0	0	0	0	0
Ovary						
EFSCH	1	0	0	0	0	0
Barnes Hospital	8	1	13	62	25	25
Vulva						
EFSCH	5	2	40	60	60	20
Barnes Hospital	3	0	0	66	33	33
Vagina						
EFSCH	10	2	20	70	56	56
Barnes Hospital	13	1	8	77	38	38
Anus						
EFSCH	1	0	0	0	0	0
Barnes Hospital	2	0	0	0	0	0
Small intestine						
EFSCH	–	–	–	–	–	–
Barnes Hospital	2	0	0	100	50	0
Bartholin's gland						
EFSCH	1	0	0	0	0	0
Barnes Hospital	–	–	–	–	–	–
Radiation necrosis, pelvic viscera						
EFSCH	0	–	–	–	–	–
Barnes Hospital	13	3	23	69	61	61
Prostate						
EFSCH	1	0	0	100	100	0
Barnes Hospital	1	1	100	0	0	0
Fibrosarcoma, iliac bone						
EFSCH	1	0	0	0	0	0

*All accumulative survival rates were calculated according to the method described in the statistical appendix.

1965). Otherwise, there would be a risk of having lymph which contained cancer cells leak into the intrapelvic wound.

CERVIX UTERI

The most frequent indication for exenterative surgery of the pelvis is carcinoma of the cervix uteri which has recurred after radiation therapy. These cancers are the most biologically and anatomically suitable for exenteration and occur with the greatest frequency. Among 172 radical pelvic operations performed at the EFSCH, 65 were for carcinomas of the cervix, while 50 were done for carcinoma of the bladder (Table 3–1). The frequency of carcinoma of the cervix as an operative indication in the Barnes Hospital series was higher because the Bricker-Butcher series is a referral series largely excluding bladder cancers (Table 3–2).

The experience at Barnes Hospital also shows cervical carcinoma persistent or recurrent after irradiation to be the most clearly defined indication for exenteration of the pelvic organs. Only 3 of the 209 women who underwent pelvic exenteration for carcinoma of the cer-

Table 3–2 Exenteration of Pelvic Organs for
Advanced Pelvic Carcinoma from 1950 to 1965 at Barnes Hospital*

INDICATIONS	NUMBER OF PATIENTS	OPERATIVE MORTALITY	5-YEAR SURVIVAL RATE (BASED ON THOSE AT RISK 5 YEARS)
A. Postirradiational carcinoma of cervix	207	16 (8%)	35%
B. Carcinoma of			
1. Rectum or sigmoid	43	7 (16%)	30%
2. Endometrium	12	2 (17%)	
3. Vagina	13	1 (8%)	
4. Bladder or urethra	6	0	
5. Ovary	8	1 (13%)	
6. Vulva or anus	5	0	
7. Small bowel	2	0	
C. Sarcoma of the prostate	1	1	
D. Palliative operations for cancer of cervix	2	1	
E. Irradiation necrosis	13	3 (23%)	
Total	312	32 (10%)	

*From Kiselow, M., Butcher, H. R., Jr., and Bricker, E. M.: Results of the radical surgical treatment of advanced pelvic cancer: a fifteen-year study. Ann. Surg., *166*:428, 1967.

vix had not had radiation therapy; a few others had been previously treated by both radiation and surgery. Some of the women had received inadequate initial radiation therapy, but were not considered for further radiation treatment because of the extent of the lesion and the presence of some persistent tissue changes caused by radiation. On the other hand, many patients had been treated unsuccessfully for their recurrence by further radiation and were referred for possible pelvic exenteration in the final stages of their disease. The factor common to all patients was the presence of carcinoma of the cervix, either persistent after adequate radiation therapy or of such advanced degree that the chance of cure without pelvic exenteration was considered negligible. An examination of Tables 3–3 and 3–4 shows that the lesions frequently invaded the bladder, rectum, pelvic soft tissues, blood vessels and nerve sheaths. Lymph node metastases were less frequent. In view of the extent of the lesions found by pathological examination and the uncertainty of determining the extent by physical examination, total pelvic exenteration has become the procedure of choice. Only in the occasional patient is the lesion sufficiently high and anterior in the pelvis to allow the rectal stump and levator muscles to be preserved safely. Lesions suitable for posterior exenteration with preservation of ureters and bladder function are not seen in patients with advanced persistent cervical carcinoma.

Pelvic exenteration has also been performed for cervical carcinoma recurrent in the central pelvis after previous hysterectomy. Daniel and Brunschwig reported 28 total and five anterior exenterations for this indication, and seven patients lived over five years (Daniel).

Table 3–3   Pathological Findings in the Operative Specimens of 19 Women Surviving Five or More Years after Pelvic Exenteration[*]

LOCATION OF CARCINOMA[**]	NO. OF PATIENTS
Soft tissue (parametrium)	17
Cervix (limited to cervix in 1)	14
Vagina	13
Bladder (preoperative hydronephrosis in 4)	12
Nerve sheaths	12
Uterus	8
Rectum	5
Vein invasion (two had external iliac vein resection)	4
Lymph nodes	2
Ileum	1

[*]From Bricker, E. M., Butcher, H. R., Jr., Lawler, W. H., Jr., and McAfee, C. A.: Surgical treatment of advanced and recurrent cancer of the pelvic viscera: an evaluation of 10 years experience. Ann. Surg., *152*:388, 1960.
[**]Epidermoid carcinoma in 15; adenocarcinoma of the cervix in 4.

Table 3–4   The Relationship of Extent of Carcinoma of the Cervix in Operative Specimens to Survival of Patients Treated by Pelvic Exenteration After Three or More Years[*]

LOCATION OF CARCINOMA	NUMBER OF PATIENTS	NUMBER OF PATIENTS DEAD OF CARCINOMA	NUMBER OF PATIENTS LIVING OR DEAD WITHOUT CARCINOMA	CHI SQUARE	PROBABILITY (a = b)
Lymph nodes					
(a) Yes	28	22	6		
(b) No	88	44	44	7.07	0.01
Blood vessels					
(a) Yes	55	38	17		
(b) No	61	28	33	6.34	0.01
Rectum or colon					
(a) Yes	35	26	9		
(b) No	81	40	41	6.18	0.01
Urinary bladder					
(a) Yes	59	40	19		
(b) No	57	26	31	5.82	0.02
Pelvic soft tissue					
(a) Yes	97	59	38		
(b) No	19	7	12	3.73	0.06
Nerve sheaths					
(a) Yes	65	42	23		
(b) No	51	24	27	3.59	0.06
Uterus					
(a) Yes	49	32	17		
(b) No	67	34	33	2.45	0.15
Vagina					
(a) Yes	90	53	37		
(b) No	26	13	13	0.65	0.4
Cervix					
(a) Yes	87	51	36		
(b) No	29	15	14	0.42	0.5
Total	116	66	50		

[*]From Kiselow, M., Butcher, H. R., Jr., and Bricker, E. M.: Results of the radical surgical treatment of advanced pelvic cancer: a fifteen-year study. Ann. Surg., *166*:428, 1967.

At the EFSCH, adenocarcinoma of the cervix uteri has been an indication for pelvic exenteration in seven cases. Three were long-term survivors (Sala).

Inoperability is determined by the demonstration of tumor outside the pelvis on physical and x-ray examinations. These findings are confirmed by biopsy when it can be done simply. The most frequently demonstrable sites of remote metastases are the lungs and the cervical and inguinal lymph nodes. The presence of physical signs of advanced disease on one side of the pelvis associated with sciatic nerve pain and swelling of the leg on the same side has proven to be a sign of inoperability. Ipsilateral ureteral obstruction at the pelvic brim is further indication of a hopeless situation. The only exceptions have been rare cases in which pelvic exenteration en bloc with hemipelvectomy was required to remove the cancer.

The intra-abdominal findings indicating inoperability are metastases to the liver, periaortic lymph nodes or extrapelvic peritoneum and such extension of the cancer within the pelvis that its complete removal is considered impossible. Deliberate palliative operations in which gross tumor is left in the pelvis are rarely indicated, having been done only twice in the patients treated at Barnes Hospital (Table 3–2). Determination of operability within the pelvis may be very difficult because radiation fibrosis and necrosis often cannot be differentiated from carcinoma by inspection and palpation. Apparent total fixation to the lateral pelvic wall does not indicate inoperability unless the fixation is due to direct carcinomatous invasion. Extent of this nature may be impossible to determine with certainty at the operating table and may become apparent only after subsequent microscopic examination of the excised specimen. Diffuse lymphatic permeation over the iliac vessels with thickening of the peritoneum and multiple underlying lymph node metastases is easily recognized and is associated frequently with leg swelling and ureteral obstruction at the pelvic brim. Such cancer dissemination is a contraindication to the operation except for the rare case manageable by en bloc hemipelvectomy. However, discrete external iliac or internal iliac lymph node metastases are not necessarily inoperable. Several patients with localized lymph node metastases attached to the iliac blood vessels have benefited significantly by resection; one such patient has lived without symptoms more than five years after her operation. Decisions concerning the operability of extensive lesions that appear still limited to the pelvis will be reflected in the mortality and survival statistics. The operability or inoperability of such lesions becomes a matter of judgment, supplemented by the frozen section examination of biopsies. Proof of inoperability is essential. Two general principles have evolved which should not be violated: (1) if persistent cancer has been proven by biopsy to exist, pelvic exenteration is not performed if it is apparent that the operation cannot remove all gross cancer; or (2) in the absence of biopsies containing cancer, the operation is not performed unless the disability of the patient from radiation fibrosis and necrosis alone warrants the procedure. For example, pelvic exenteration is sometimes justified if the lesion is associated with extensive pain, sloughing and fistula formation even though no cancer is found in the operative specimen.

Factors other than those directly related to the pathology of the neoplasm may influence operability. The general condition, age and mental status of the patient should be considered carefully. The patient must have a reasonable chance of surviving the operation and must subsequently be capable of enjoying a comfortable and useful life. Such requirements will rule out the senile and mentally deficient. Fortunately, the occasional patient who cannot adjust emotionally to the change created by pelvic exenteration usually refuses the operation when it is explained and recommended.

The survival of women who have been treated by pelvic exenteration for persistent postirradiational cancer of the uterine cervix is shown in Tables 3–1 and 3–2. Fifty-three of 153 women operated upon five or more years ago at Barnes have remained alive without signs of persistent cancer. The five-year accumulative survival rate for the entire group of women who underwent the operation for cancer of the cervix uteri was 39 per cent at Barnes and 42 per cent at EFSCH (Table 3–1). Whether this survival was the result of patient selection for the operation or represented a significant improvement in the treatment of women with persistent postirradiational cervical carcinoma was investigated by studying the survival of similarly ill women who were not treated by pelvic exenteration.

The records of all patients with cancer of the cervix seen for the first time in the Barnes Hospital from January 2, 1950 to January 1,

Table 3–5 A Comparison of (A) the Rates of Survival of Women Treated for Persistent Carcinoma by Abdominal Exploration and Exenteration of the Pelvic Organs when Operable with (B) the Rates of Survival of Those Women Having Similar Disease but Treated by Other Means[*]

MONTHS AT RISK	NUMBER OF PATIENTS		NUMBER OF PATIENTS DEAD	NUMBER OF PATIENTS ALIVE	CHI SQUARE	P A = B
0–12	(A)	138	69	69		
	(B)	118	73	45	3.64	0.07
13–24	(A)	68	22	46		
	(B)	40	22	18	5.37	0.02
25–36	(A)	45[**]	11	34		
	(B)	17[**]	9	8	4.49	0.04
37–48	(A)	31	4	27		
	(B)	8	5	3	8.82	0.005
49–60	(A)	20	4	16		
	(B)	3	1	2	–	–
60+	(A)	14	1	13		
	(B)	2	1	1	–	–

[*]From Bricker, E. M., Butcher, H. R., Jr., Lawler, W. H., Jr., and McAfee, C. A.: Surgical treatment of advanced and recurrent cancer of the pelvic viscera, and evaluation of 10 years experience. Ann. Surg., 152:388, 1960.

[**]Comparing the survival of patients three years after treatment in group A with that in group B, chi square = 14.1. Probability less than .001.

1957 were reviewed, and the diagnosis was confirmed by reexamination of their tissue sections. The initial therapy of these women had been administered in other hospitals or was given during this time at Barnes Hospital. The radiation therapy failed to eradicate the cancer in 459 out of 805 women; 256 of them might have had abdominal exploration for exenteration of the pelvis during their course as treatment for persistent cancer (Table 3–5). In other words, their persistent cancer was, for a time, apparently limited to the pelvis. Actually, 138 women had abdominal exploration and 80 had pelvic exenterations performed during this time. The remaining 118 patients included 20 who refused the operation when it was recommended to them and 8 who were not offered the operation by their physician. Further radiation was used to treat these women for their persistent cancer. Only those patients were included whose records contained sufficient data to indicate that abdominal exploration for possible pelvic exenteration was applicable as therapy for their persistent cancer.

The comparisons of the rates of survival among the 138 women undergoing abdominal exploration for pelvic exenteration (operative series) with those of the 118 women treated for persistent cancer by other means (control series) are summarized in Table 3–5 and Figure 3–9. The survival rates for the group explored for possible exenteration were significantly higher than they were for the women not so treated at each "at risk" period. The mortality rates of the patients found to have intra-abdominal cancer outside the pelvis were slightly higher than those of the control group, but not significantly so.

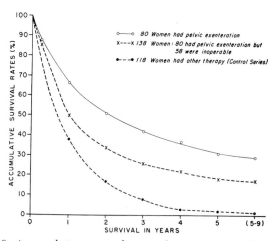

Figure 3–9 Accumulative survival rates of women treated for postirradiational cancer of the cervix at Barnes Hospital from 1950 to 1957. (From Bricker, E. M., Butcher, H. R., Jr., Lawler, W. H., Jr., and McAfee, C. A.: Surgical treatment of advanced and recurrent cancer of the pelvic viscera, an evaluation of 10 years' experience. Ann. Surg., *152*:388, 1960.)

The next question was whether or not the two groups of women were comparable (Bricker, 1960). The women in both groups had a similar incidence of adenocarcinoma of the endocervix, similar durations of symptoms and a like frequency of biopsy-proven persistent cancer at the time they were amenable to abdominal exploration for possible pelvic exenteration. However, the age distribution of the two groups differed. The women undergoing abdominal exploration for possible pelvic exenteration were younger than those not so treated. This is to be expected, particularly among the earlier cases of the group treated operatively, because initially the older women were not considered eligible for pelvic exenteration since the operative risk was thought to be excessive. Since age alone has been shown not to influence the survival of women treated for cancer of the cervix, the effect of the difference in age distribution upon the survival of patients in the two groups can be calculated from statistical tables showing the overall expected mortality rates of all women. Only an additional 3 per cent of the women in the control group would be expected to die from all causes during a five-year period than in the group explored for possible pelvic exenteration. In other words, the divergence of the age distribution of the two groups of women does not account for the difference in their survival rates.

The control and operative series also differed in the distribution of women by the initial clinical stage of their cancers. The stages of the cancer in women undergoing abdominal exploration for pelvic exenteration were significantly more advanced than in the women treated by other means (control series). This difference might be expected to reduce the length of the survival of the women undergoing surgery. The data are inadequate to allow an estimate of this reduction. Its direction, however, is opposite that resulting from the difference in age distributions of the two groups of women. One then may conclude logically that the survival rates of the women treated operatively for persistent cancer were higher because their treatment was more effective.

The extent of cancer in the operative specimens of patients surviving three or more years was representative of the advanced stage of disease that characterized the majority of lesions (Table 3–4). It is of interest that two patients with regional lymph node metastases and two patients requiring external iliac vein resection are among these survivors. Of the patients dying of recurrent cancer after exenteration, approximately 75 per cent had recurrence in the pelvis. The remainder died of metastasis to liver, lungs, bone or brain.

At the EFSCH, coordination of primary therapy and follow-up with the radiation therapist was possible more frequently (Gary). Among 554 consecutive new cervix cancer cases staged and treated primarily by radiotherapy at the EFSCH from 1950 to 1959, 299 cancers were not controlled. Fourteen of these (5 per cent) were salvaged either by additional radiotherapy to discrete vaginal recurrences or by pelvic exenteration. Based on observed progression of cancer in the pelvis, we estimate that at least 9 per cent of these failures could have been salvaged by earlier detection and pelvic exenteration.

URINARY BLADDER

The bladder wall is quite thin, and invasive bladder cancers extend into the perivesical fat when the primary cancer may still be relatively small. This fat lies between the visceral and parietal layer of pelvic fascia. Also, bladder cancers seem to be highly implantable in open wounds. The only plane available for dissection that would avoid transecting cancer which extended into the perivesical fat lies between the parietal layer of pelvic fascia and the musculoskeletal pelvis. Exenterative dissection in this plane probably negates the curative value of simple cystectomy for invasive bladder cancers whose greatest chordal dimension as viewed through a cystoscope is more than twice the thickness of the bladder wall.

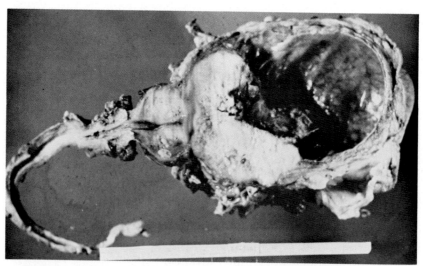

Figure 3–10 Specimen resulting from the abdominoperineal resection of the urethra, prostate and bladder combined with intrapelvic mobilization of the bladder by dissecting between the parietal layer of endopelvic fascia and the musculoskeletal wall of the pelvis. (From Long, R. T. L., Grummon, R. A., Spratt, J. S., Jr., and Perez-Mesa, C.: Carcinoma of the urinary bladder [comparison with radical, simple and partial cystectomy and intravesical formalin]. Cancer, *29*:98, 1972.)

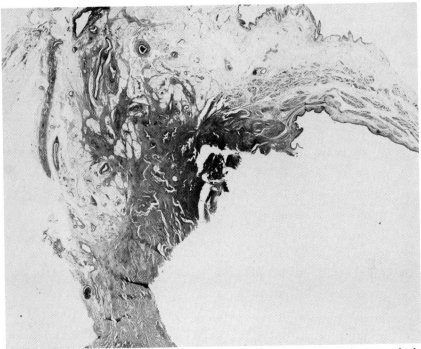

Figure 3–11 Invasion of relatively small bladder cancers through the entire thickness of the bladder wall into the perivesical fat is an important characteristic in dictating the type of operation to be performed. To remove the invaded fat without exposing or transecting occult cancer, the bladder must be removed en bloc with its fatty areolar envelope by dissecting between the parietal layer of the endopelvic fascia and the musculoskeletal wall of the pelvis. The perivesical fat is contained between the visceral layer of endopelvic fascia adjacent to the bladder and the parietal endopelvic fascia. (From Long, R. T. L., Grummon, R. A., Spratt, J. S., Jr., and Perez-Mesa, C.: Carcinoma of the urinary bladder [comparison with radical, simple and partial cystectomy and intravesical formalin]. Cancer, 29:98, 1972.)

Long, Grummon, Spratt and Perez-Mesa conducted a clinical management review of the entire experience with bladder cancer seen at the EFSCH and the CRC between 1940 and 1971 and reported the experience with resective surgery (Long, 1971). The results clearly establish that abdominoperineal radical cystectomy coupled with the use of intravesical and intraurethral formalin as a precaution against implantation metastases gives superior results for invasive neoplasms.

Figures 3–10 and 3–11 show the gross morphology of a typical bladder cancer. The cancer extended through the bladder wall and into the perivesical fat. It did not transgress the parietal layer of pelvic fascia, and it had not metastasized to regional lymph nodes in spite of its size and local extension. This bladder was removed by a radical abdominoperineal cystectomy and urethrectomy en bloc. The end re-

Table 3–6   End Results Attending Resective Surgery for Bladder Cancer by Grade, 1940–1971*

Type of Operation	Grade	No. of Cases	Accumulative Survival Rate (%), Age Adjusted			Accumulative Survival Rate (%) with Standard Deviation (No Age Adjustment)		
			1 yr.	3 yrs.	5 yrs.	1 yr.	3 yrs.	5 yrs.
Partial cystectomy	1	10	100	100	100	100 ± 0	100 ± 0	90 ± 9
	2	9	92	38	38	89 ± 10	33 ± 16	33 ± 16
	3	13	89	27	27	85 ± 10	23 ± 12	23 ± 12
	4	8	90	26	14	88 ± 12	25 ± 15	13 ± 12
	Unknown	2	100	0	0	100 ± 0	0	0
		42						
Simple cystectomy, no lymph node dissection	1	17	91	79	62	88 ± 8	71 ± 11	53 ± 12
	2	17	49	19	19	47 ± 12	18 ± 9	18 ± 9
	3	14	60	17	17	57 ± 13	14 ± 9	14 ± 9
	4	4	0	0	0	0	0	0
	Unknown	3	100	74	74	100 ± 0	67 ± 27	67 ± 27
		55						
Radical supralevator cystectomy with lymph nodes	1	6	87	72	72	83 ± 15	67 ± 19	67 ± 19
	2	5	62	21	21	60 ± 22	20 ± 18	20 ± 18
	3	5	42	42	0	40 ± 22	40 ± 22	0
	4	4	26	26	0	25 ± 22	25 ± 22	0
	Unknown	0	0	0	0	0	0	0
		20						
Radical cystectomy, prostatectomy and urethrectomy	1	5	63	63	63	60 ± 22	60 ± 22	60 ± 22
	2	5	64	64	64	60 ± 22	60 ± 22	60 ± 22
	3	13	80	69	69	77 ± 12	61 ± 14	61 ± 14
	4	11	54	44	25	52 ± 15	41 ± 16	20 ± 16
	Unknown	0	0	0	0	0	0	0
		34						
Radical abdomino- perineal cys- tectomy, no lymph nodes in specimen	1	3	35	35	35	33 ± 27	33 ± 27	33 ± 27
	2	1	0	0	0	0	0	0
	3	1	100	0	0	100 ± 0	0	0
	4	2	52	52	52	50 ± 35	50 ± 0	50 ± 0
	Unknown	0	0	0	0	0	0	0
		7						
	Total	158						

*From Long, R. T. L., Grummon, R. A., Spratt, J. S., Jr., and Perez-Mesa, C.: Carcinoma of the urinary bladder (comparison with radical, simple, and partial cystectomy and intravesical formalin). Cancer, 29:98, 1972.

sults for bladder cancer by operation, stage and grade seen consecutively at the EFSCH between 1940 and 1971 are given in Tables 3–6 and 3–7.

During the 1940–1971 period, sufficient radiotherapy was always available at the EFSCH. However, radiotherapy was not well tolerated by the patients treated, usually because of the advanced stage of the cancers and associated sepsis. No experience has accumulated with recent trends in performing a urinary diversion followed by radiotherapy.

Table 3–7 End Results Attending Resective Surgery for Bladder Cancer by Jewett's Staging, 1940–1971[*]

Type of Operation	Stage	No. of Cases	Accumulative Survival Rate (%), Age Adjusted			Accumulative Survival Rate (%) with Standard Deviation (No Age Adjustment)		
			1 yr.	3 yrs.	5 yrs.	1 yr.	3 yrs.	5 yrs.
Partial cystectomy	0	5	100	100	86	100 ± 0	100 ± 0	80 ± 18
	A	6	100	75	75	100 ± 0	67 ± 19	67 ± 19
	B_1	7	89	48	48	86 ± 13	43 ± 19	43 ± 19
	B_2	5	100	23	23	100 ± 0	20 ± 18	20 ± 18
	B_1 or B_2	4	76	26	0	75 ± 22	25 ± 22	0
	C	11	87	11	11	82 ± 12	9 ± 9	9 ± 9
	D	1	100	0	0	100 ± 0	0	0
	Unknown	3	100	100	100	100 ± 0	100 ± 0	100 ± 0
		42						
Simple cystectomy, no lymph node dissection	0	11	85	49	21	82 ± 12	45 ± 15	18 ± 12
	A	8	100	100	100	100 ± 0	88 ± 12	88 ± 12
	B_1	1	100	0	0	100 ± 0	0	0
	B_2	6	86	55	55	83 ± 15	50 ± 20	50 ± 20
	B_1 or B_2	6	51	18	18	50 ± 20	17 ± 15	17 ± 15
	C	20	36	11	11	35 ± 11	10 ± 7	10 ± 7
	D	2	0	0	0	0	0	0
	Unknown	1	100	100	100	100 ± 0	100 ± 0	100 ± 0
		55						
Radical supralevator cystectomy with lymph nodes	0	2	100	100	100	100 ± 0	100 ± 0	100 ± 0
	A	1	100	100	100	100 ± 0	100 ± 0	100 ± 0
	B_2	1	100	0	0	100 ± 0	0	0
	B_1 or B_2	2	0	0	0	0	0	0
	C	7	45	16	16	43 ± 19	14 ± 13	14 ± 0
	D	6	52	52	20	50 ± 20	50 ± 20	17 ± 15
	Unknown	1	100	100	100	100 ± 0	100 ± 0	100 ± 0
		20						
Radical cystectomy, prostatectomy, and urethrectomy	0	3	69	69	69	67 ± 27	67 ± 27	67 ± 27
	A	5	82	82	82	80 ± 18	80 ± 18	80 ± 18
	B_1	4	80	80	80	75 ± 22	75 ± 22	75 ± 22
	B_2	4	27	27	27	25 ± 22	25 ± 0	25 ± 0
	B_1 or B_2	3	69	36	36	67 ± 27	33 ± 27	33 ± 27
	C	10	72	51	51	68 ± 15	44 ± 17	44 ± 17
	D	5	62	62	24	60 ± 22	60 ± 22	20 ± 24
	Unknown	0						
		34						
Radical abdomino-perineal cys-tectomy, no lymph nodes in specimen	0	3	35	35	35	33 ± 27	33 ± 27	33 ± 27
	C	4	51	0	0	50 ± 25	0	0
		7						
Total		158						

[*]From Long, R. T. L., Grummon, R. A., Spratt, J. S., Jr. and Perez-Mesa, C.: Carcinoma of the urinary bladder (comparison with radical, simple, and partial cystectomy and intravesical formalin). Cancer, 29:98, 1972.

RECTUM AND PELVIC COLON

The indications for exenterative surgery for colorectal carcinomas is encountered in a minority of cases. However, there exists a biological type of adenocarcinoma of the colorectum that can exhibit progressive local growth and extend through the bowel wall into adjacent pericolic fat and contiguous viscera, such as that of the prostate, bladder, uterus, small intestine and vagina. In spite of the great local size and extension, these cancers remain localized, spreading to neither lymph nodes, liver nor other sites. They are often associated with expanding or well-circumscribed margins and intense inflammation, including microscopic abscesses (Spratt, 1970). These cancers may even perforate and develop fistulas while still remaining localized (Sperling). Also, certain colorectal cancers that do metastasize to lymph nodes may have metastases restricted to only a few lymph nodes in immediate proximity to the cancer. Of 11 exenteration specimens which contained lymph node metastases, only two patients had more than two lymph nodes involved (Butcher).

Previous observations on the natural history of colorectal neoplasms give an explanation as to why patients tolerate the presence of such large, localized visceral cancers before coming to a physician. Adenocarcinomas of the colorectum grow very slowly in many instances, as measured by serial roentgen observations (Welin). In fact, some grow so slowly that they are present for many years before they are discovered. Discovery is often incidental to the development of obstruction, perforation or bleeding. In many cases, the patients will have a history suggesting longstanding partial obstruction. The obstruction rarely becomes complete before the cancer has invaded the outer muscular layer of the intestinal wall. This layer is responsible for the opening wave of peristalsis (Ragland). Indeed, in many of these cases the neoplasm extends beyond the bowel wall into contiguous structures. Any surgeon exploring a patient with a large colorectal cancer with symptoms of partial obstruction should be prepared to perform multiple organ resections and pelvic exenteration when necessary for the complete removal of the primary cancer.

Rare indications reported in the literature but not included in the EFSCH and Barnes Hospital experience will be discussed for completeness. These include sarcoma botryoides (Parsons) and sarcoma of the ovary. Ovarian cancer often extends beyond the pelvic confines. Long and Sala reported 17 surgically treated advanced ovarian cancers. Three had multiorgan resections with long-term control of the cancer in only one case (Long and Sala, 1963). Only one patient at the EFSCH had an exenteration for prostate cancer. Urethral cancers are amenable to resective surgery occasionally. Four exenterations have been done for urethral cancer at the EFSCH and Barnes Hospital, two at each institution. Grabstald reported nine anterior exenterations and one total exenteration for cancer of the female urethra. Of these, three were long-term survivors (Grabstald).

VAGINA

Masterson, Sala and Spratt reported two patients who had pelvic exenterations for epidermoid vaginal cancer who survived 27 and 64 months (Masterson). Advanced age of the patients and the infrequency of vaginal cancer keep the indications for exenteration low. At the present time, eight total exenterations and two anterior exenterations have been performed for vaginal cancer at the EFSCH. Five of the eight were alive and free of disease 16 months to six years after total procedure. One of the two persons having an anterior exenteration is alive and free of disease four and one-half years after resection, and the other patient lived 26 months after the procedure. One postoperative death occurred among the ten patients (10 per cent).

Smith reported three total exenterations for vaginal cancer (Smith). One patient was free of disease at the third postoperative year, but the other two developed recurrent cancer and died. Five partial exenterations were also reported by Smith, and two of these patients were long-term survivors.

VULVA

When carcinoma of the vulva advances to involve the urethra, vagina, anus and/or rectum, it may require en bloc pelvic exenteration and radical vulvectomy to insure total extirpation of the cancer. Of course, the indication for this operation does not occur often. However, Brunschwig and Daniel reported 27 patients so treated (Brunschwig). Sixteen required only anterior exenterations. His operative mortality was 57 per cent. Only two patients could be classified as long-term survivors (eight years). Green, Uhlfelder and Meigs reported results with 238 cases of epidermoid cancer of the vulva (Green). Of these, three patients underwent posterior pelvic exenteration without hospital mortality. Two of the three patients died eight and 13 years later. Symmonds, Pratt and Dockerty reported an anterior exenteration and delayed bilateral groin dissection for melanoma of the vulva with positive involvement of lymph nodes (Symmonds). The patient survived more than four years, later dying of causes not related to the melanoma.

Sites of miscellaneous lesions for which exenterative surgery of the pelvis has been performed include urethra, Bartholin's greater vestibular glands, ovaries, prostate, primary small intestinal cancers invading pelvic structures secondarily, and musculoskeletal sarcomas of the pelvis invading or compressing pelvic viscera (Table 3–1). Generally, the results obtained with these lesions have been poor. There are, however, exceptions. Each infrequent neoplasm must be separately evaluated regarding anatomical extent and biological behavior. Occasional neoplasms can occur in almost any pelvic tissue if they have the biological propensity to remain localized, though they may obtain extensive local growth involving one or more pelvic viscera, including the musculoskeletal pelvis. If a biologically favorable lesion is anatomically situated as to permit encompassing exenterative surgery, the procedure may be worthwhile from the standpoints of both cure and palliation.

RADIATION NECROSIS

The effect of radiation on living tissue is a function of a number of factors including host tolerance, location and extent of the original neoplasm, sensitivity of the neoplasm, variations in the size and shape of the host, associated illnesses and infections, a host of physical variables specific to the type of ionizing radiation utilized, time of administration and calculated distribution of the dose. With such a variety of factors affecting the outcome, isolated or more generalized areas of poorly tolerated treatment may result. The later problems in the host come from degree of damage to normal tissue, which is both general and specific. The faster growing tissues, such as intestinal mucosa and bone marrow, are among the most sensitive. Endothelium in blood vessels and lymphatics is quite sensitive. However, all tissues are affected to varying degrees by direct cellular death which is somewhat randomly distributed throughout the tissues and by ischemia secondary to vascular injury. Initially, damaged cells are absorbed and partially replaced by regeneration and scar. The capacity to regenerate is a function of time-dose factors characterizing the radiation and of the resulting partial ischemia.

When the endothelia of blood vessels and lymphatics are sufficiently damaged, capillary budding requisite for the formation of granulation tissue and normal wound healing is retarded. Consequently, tissues which have been heavily radiated or which are unusually sensitive to injury may develop progressive necrosis and little healing. When this process starts in the pelvis it may progress through mucosal ulceration and increasing organ necrosis. We have called this problem the "cloacal syndrome." The unfortunate victims of this syndrome require well understood and carefully planned treatment, for the pitfalls that can compound patient morbidity are many.

Fortunately, the radiation necrosis of pelvic organs is not a frequent indication for pelvic exenteration. However, when such is the case, exenteration may be lifesaving. When radiation ulcers of the urinary bladder or rectum exist, and when vesicovaginal or rectovaginal fistulas have occurred, simple diversionary procedures may suffice (Sugg). When subsequent healing fails to occur and progressive necrosis and infection develop, removal of all pelvic organs damaged by the radiation and complicating infection is indicated.

Considerable judgment is required in the selection of the patients injured by radiation who will be candidates for exenterative surgery. If this procedure is too long delayed, the persistent necrosis and infection may produce such cachexia and inanition that exenteration cannot be physiologically tolerated. Such was the case in two of the three patients who died postoperatively (Table 3–2).

PELVIC EXENTERATION AS PRIMARY THERAPY FOR ADVANCED STAGE CANCERS OF THE CERVIX UTERI

Ketcham et al. and Deckers and Ketcham et al. also reported a growing experience with the use of pelvic exenteration as the primary treatment for selected stage III and IV carcinomas of the cervix uteri. An accumulative five-year survival rate of 48.5 per cent in 65 patients was achieved. The presence of metastatic carcinoma in the pelvic lymph nodes did not affect prognosis adversely. Careful preoperative evaluation and intraoperative exploratory evaluation were mandatory for these patients in order to exclude the presence of extrapelvic disease. The authors concluded that their experience merited more frequent consideration of pelvic exenteration as primary therapy for selected cancers of the cervix uteri.

LATE SECOND PRIMARY CANCERS IN THE PELVIS

Women who have had radiation therapy for carcinoma of the cervix uteri are also at risk to develop late second primary cancer. Deckers and Sugarbaker et al. recently reported 18 genital second primary cancers occurring 7 to 20 years after radiotherapy to an epidermoid cancer of the cervix uteri. The second cancers were usually large and locally destructive at the time of discovery, though they had produced symptoms for a relatively short period of time. All were treated by pelvic exenteration, attaining a 35 per cent five-year accumulative survival rate. The surgical mortality rate was high in this group (6 of 18 cases, or 33 per cent). The authors attributed this high mortality rate to the complications attending pelvic exenterations in irradiated pelves.

REFERENCES

Bricker, E. M., Butcher, H. R., Jr., Lawler, W. H., Jr., and McAfee, C. A.: Surgical treatment of advanced and recurrent cancer of the pelvic viscera, an evaluation of 10 years experience. Ann. Surg., 152:388, 1960.

Butcher, H. R., Jr., and Spjut, H. J.: An evaluation of pelvic exenteration for advanced carcinoma of the lower colon. Cancer, 12:681, 1959.

Brunschwig, A., and Daniel, W.: Pelvic exenterations for advanced carcinoma of the vulva. Am. J. Obstet. Gynecol., 72:489, 1956.

Daniel, W. W., and Brunschwig, A.: The management of recurrent carcinoma of the cervix following simple total hysterectomy. Cancer, 14:582, 1961.

Deckers, P. J., Ketcham, A. S., Sugarbaker, E. V., Hoye, R. C., and Thomas, L. B.: Pelvic exenteration for primary carcinoma of the uterine cervix. Obstet. Gynecol., 37:647, 1971.

Deckers, P. J., Sugarbaker, E. V., Pilch, Y. H., and Ketcham, A. S.: Pelvic exenteration for late second cancers of the uterine cervix after earlier irradiation. Ann. Surg., 175:48, 1972.

Dillard, B. M., Spratt, J. S., Jr., Ackerman, L. V., and Butcher, H. R., Jr.: Epidermoid cancer of anal margin and canal. Arch. Surg., 86:772, 1963.

Gary, R. K., Sala, J. M., and Spratt, J. S., Jr.: The detection and treatment of postirradiationally recidivated cancers of the cervix uteri. Radiology, 83:208, 1964.

Grabstald, H., Hilaris, B., Henschke, U., and Whitmore, W. F., Jr.: Cancer of the female urethra. J.A.M.A., 197:835, 1966.

Green, T. H., Jr., Ulfelder, H., and Meigs, J. V.: Epidermoid carcinoma of the vulva: an analysis of 238 cases. Am. J. Obstet. Gynecol., 75:834, 1958.

Ketcham, A. S., Deckers, P. J., Sugarbaker, E. V., Hoye, R. C., Thomas, L. B., and Smith, R. R.: Pelvic exenteration for carcinoma of the uterine cervix, a 15-year experience. Cancer, 26:513, 1970.

Long, R. T. L., and Sala, J. M.: Radical pelvic surgery combined with radiotherapy in the treatment of locally advanced ovarian carcinoma. Surg. Gynecol. Obstet., 117:201, 1963.

Long, R. T. L., Grummon, R. A., Spratt, J. S., Jr., and Perez-Mesa, C.: Carcinoma of the urinary bladder (comparison with radical, simple and partial cystectomy and intravesical formalin). Cancer, 29:98, 1972.

Masterson, B. J., Sala, J. M., and Spratt, J. S., Jr.: Epidermoid carcinoma of the vagina. Mo. Med., 59:1182, 1962.

Ragland, J. J., Londe, A. M., and Spratt, J. S., Jr.: Correlation of the prognosis of obstructing colorectal carcinoma with clinical and pathologic variables. Am. J. Surg., 121:552, 1971.

Sala, J. M., Gleason, J. A., and Spratt, J. S., Jr.: Adenocarcinoma of the cervix uteri. Mo. Med., 59:1168, 1962.

Smith, F. R.: Primary carcinoma of vagina. Am. J. Obstet. Gynecol., 69:525, 1955.

Sperling, D., Spratt, J. S., Jr., and Carnes, V. M.: Adenocarcinoma of the large intestine with perforation. Mo. Med., 60:1104, 1963.

Spratt, J. S., Jr.: The log normal frequency distribution and human cancer. J. Surg. Res., 9:151, 1969.

Spratt, J. S., Jr., Shieber, W., and Dillard, B. M.: Anatomy and Surgical Technique of Groin Dissection. Saint Louis, The C. V. Mosby Co., 1965.

Spratt, J. S., Jr., and Spratt, T. L.: Correlation of the rates of growth of pulmonary metastases and host survival. Ann. Surg., 159:161, 1964.

Spratt, J. S., Jr., Watson, F. R., and Pratt, J. L.: Characteristics of a variant of colorectal carcinoma that do not metastasize to lymph nodes. Dis. Colon Rectum, 13:243, 1970.

Sugg, W. L., Lawler, W. H., Ackerman, L. V., and Butcher, H. R., Jr.: Operative therapy for severe irradiational injury in the enteral and urinary tracts. Ann. Surg., 157:62, 1963.

Symmonds, R. E., Pratt, J. H., and Dockerty, M. B.: Melanoma of the vulva. Obstet. Gynecol., 15:543, 1960.

Welin, S., Youker, J., and Spratt, J. S., Jr.: The rates and patterns of growth of 375 tumors of the large intestine and rectum observed serially by double contrast enema study (Malmo technique). Am. J. Roentgenol. Radium Ther. Nucl. Med., 90:673, 1963.

Chapter Four

PREOPERATIVE
EVALUATION

Pelvic exenteration should be considered in the following situations:

Biopsy-proven pelvic cancer of any type that is

1. Recurrent after maximum tolerable dose of radiation therapy to the midpelvis

2. Extending from the organ of origin and not a candidate for radiation therapy for any of the following reasons:

    a. Pathological type of cancer is not responsive to radiation

    b. Anatomical extent of the cancer is not amenable to radiation therapy or radiation therapy would produce fistulas

    c. Presence of intravisceral fistulas

    d. Unilateral or bilateral obstruction of the ureters as confirmed by intravenous pyelography

Patient characteristics contraindicating pelvic exenteration are

1. Rigid fixation to bony pelvis unless bone can be resected en bloc

2. Intractable unilateral sciatic pain unless hemipelvectomy with resection of the sciatic plexus can be performed en bloc

3. Medical or psychiatric contraindications to major surgery, such as

    a. Senility

    b. Neuropsychiatric disorders producing uncooperative patients who are incapable of following instructions

    c. Any medical disorder not otherwise correctable with a life expectancy of less than two years

    d. Angina pectoris, malignant hypertension, repeated or re-
cent myocardial infarctions, physically disabling pulmonary emphysema, uncontrolled cardiac failure (Moyer),
advanced renal and hepatic insufficiency (serum al-
bumin less than 3 gm. per 100 ml and BUN over 50 mg.
per 100 ml.)

    e. Uncorrectable bleeding or clotting disorders

Pelvic exenteration should not be performed when certain envi-
ronmental or manpower deficiencies exist, such as

    1. Surgical suite with inadequate instruments and a scrub team
unfamiliar with the procedure and its instruments

    2. Blood bank incapable of making six units available before
operations start and additional units on demand

    3. Anesthesiology team not cognizant of problems peculiar to
exenterative surgery, including such factors as

    a. Duration of operation

    b. Blood loss, including both volume and rate

    c. Intra-abdominal packing with potential elevation of dia-
phragms, obstruction of inferior vena cava, torsional obstruction of hepatic veins

The same preoperative evaluation of persons being considered
for exenterative surgery of the pelvis that is applied to persons being
considered for major surgery of any type must be done. The great
stress of this operation demands a good physiological reserve in all
vital systems and requires that the patient be in optimum physiological balance. Age itself is no contraindication, but many of the
problems that develop in aging persons are contraindications.

The minimum components of a preoperative evaluation include
the following:

    1. Routine history and physical examination

    2. Exact information on all previous radiation therapy, includ-
ing the location of all external radiation ports, type of radiation and
midpelvic dose (Spratt, 1962)

    3. Careful bimanual pelvic examination by the *operating
surgeon* performed under anesthesia when apprehension, pain or
obesity make an examination on an awake patient incomplete or inadequate for careful bimanual assessment of the extent of the neoplasm

    4. Histological diagnosis of persistent cancer

    5. Cystoscopic examination when bladder involvement is sus-
pected

    6. Proctoscopic examination with evaluation of colorectal in-
volvement and exclusion of second primary cancers on mucosa
viewed through proctoscope

    7. Informed consent of the patient and the immediate family

    8. Laboratory tests: urinalysis, hemogram, BUN, serum pro-

teins, creatinine, alkaline phosphatase, EKG, blood type with minimum of six cross-matched units available and additional units available on demand

9. Roentgen evaluation: chest x-ray, intravenous pyelograms, bony pelvis, roentgen evaluation of all areas producing symptoms suggestive of extrapelvic metastases

10. Blind biopsy of scalene lymph nodes (Ketcham et al., 1972)

The recent addition of the scalene node biopsy seems justified on the basis of Ketcham's observations. Ketcham has reported his experience in the performance of scalene lymph node biopsies in the evaluation of potential candidates for surgical ablation of cancer of the cervix uteri. He found that 13.5 per cent of the patients thought to have cancer of the cervix uteri restricted to the pelvis already had metastatic cancer in the scalene lymph nodes. When metastatic cancer is present in these lymph nodes on microscopic examination, obviously the cancer is no longer localized to the pelvis in spite of any clinical impression to the contrary. Unfortunately, neither the Barnes nor the EFSCH series contains data that would permit a correlation between clinical evaluation of resectability and the presence or absence of scalene lymph node metastases (Ketcham et al., 1972).

Other well-recognized contraindications to exenterative pelvic surgery exist. Mental status and attitude of the patient are very important determinants of operability. Intelligent, understanding cooperation of the patient is absolutely necessary during the postoperative and rehabilitative periods. This must include the ability of the patient to comprehend the preoperative explanation in order that informed consent can be given. Consequently, a psychoses characterized by uncooperative attitudes or senility to the point of extreme forgetfulness, disorientation and lack of concern are contraindications. The mental attitude of the patient can be affected very significantly by the surgeon's relationship with the patient. For the patient to participate fully in his rehabilitative care, he must be educated and motivated. Patient education improves cooperation, allays fears that arise from uncertainty and reduces the chances of complications arising from the patient's actions. The nature of the exenterative operation must be explained to the patient in positive, concise terms intended to attain understanding and cooperation. The most straightforward approach is to state the probabilities of permanent control based on extant experience and to emphasize the fact that long periods of productive survival can be obtained. Since the operation will terminate sexual activity, both the patient and the spouse must be informed. Patients need to understand that cancer is a chronic disease which is highly curable in many instances. Many human afflictions have a far worse and more inevitably lethal prognosis. This fact is psychologically reassuring to many people who incorrectly associate all forms of cancer with death (Cunningham).

The chronicity of the cancer and the nature of the exenterative and reconstructive aspects of the operation require systematic, long-term management to attain optimal results. The education of the patient and his family requires a systematic approach to avoid errors of omission. The job of educating the patient can be simplified by developing appropriate teaching aids covering various aspects of management such as preoperative explanations, postoperative care and follow-up. These aids should be written in concise, basic English and supplemented with appropriate illustrations. The nursing service must be thoroughly familiar with these documents, since nurses are so frequently interrogated by the patient and are necessary participants in patient and family education for appropriate care. The education may be performed by others, depending on the local system used, including health educators, enterostomal therapists, rehabilitation staff or physician's assistants.

Teaching aids can be of assistance in helping the patient to develop the proper attitude during the preoperative evaluation with continuance into the postoperative period.

EVALUATORY EXAMINATION

When an evaluatory examination is performed under general anesthesia or on the awake cooperative patient, a careful palpation of the relaxed abdomen and groin is done first. Particular attention is paid to the transabdominal periaortic palpation for renal enlargement or tenderness, to the umbilical palpation for metastases to the umbilicus and to the general abdominal palpation for other masses. The scalene and inguinal lymph nodes occasionally contain palpable metastases from cancers arising in pelvic or abdominal viscera. Many patients have palpable inguinal lymph nodes. When one or more of these nodes is disproportionately enlarged or hardened, the surgeon should perform an open excisional biopsy of the node.

For larger mobile nodes with metastases, a palliative superficial groin dissection is occasionally justified to avoid local overgrowth with femoral artery and skin invasion with resultant hemorrhage, ulceration, added nursing care and other avoidable morbidity (Spratt, 1965, p. 77). Cancers arising in the vagina, cervix, endometrium, ovary or colorectum that have inguinal metastases are with rare exception incurable by definitive surgery. An occasional cancer, however, can involve these nodes or the lateral pelvic wall and still be either curable by selected combinations of surgical procedures that will encompass all of the disease or controllable for protracted periods of symptom-free survival. As an example, among 148 patients undergoing radical groin dissections, six had cancers originating in the pelvic viscera (Spratt, 1965). A rectal cancer that recurred in the perineum with metastases to the inguinal lymph nodes after abdominoperineal resection was controlled by wide resection of the involved perineum and bilateral groin dissections.

To continue with the evaluation, the patient is placed in the lithotomy position. If biopsies are planned, the lower abdomen, perineum and vagina are prepared with alcohol Betadine, and the bladder is emptied of urine. The perineum, vulva, urethra, meatus and anus are inspected for abnormalities. Following this the bimanual palpatory examination is done. The right pelvis is generally examined with the right hand, the left pelvis with the left hand. The location, size and extent of any pelvic mass are determined. Particular attention is given to possible extensions and/or fixations of the primary cancer to other organs and to the pelvic wall. The exact anatomical sites of a fixation can be determined with some experience. When the cancer is in the cervix, particular attention is paid to the uterosacral ligaments and the parametrium. These areas are best evaluated by rectovaginal or rectal palpation. The presence or absence of palpable extension into any pelvic organ should be noted and recorded.

In examining the rectum of patients with rectal cancers, the size, fixation and degree of mobility are noted. Bimanual palpation of rectal lesions may suggest involvement of the bladder trigone, prostate or vagina. The cancer may also be fixed on the sacrum or coccyx. Cystoscopic examination is performed when bladder involvement is suspected.

Patients who have had previous pelvic radiation require special care in evaluation. First, the surgeon should know the location and size of both the entry and the exit radiation ports, the energy characteristics of the radiation and the tissue dose in the ports and to the midpelvis. With high energy radiation, such as that which comes from cobalt 50, a betatron or a linear accelerator, more tissue reaction may occur on the side of the body *opposite* the port of entry. Consequently, either entry ports or exit ports may exhibit skin changes and subcutaneous fibrosis attributable to the radiation. The palpable fibrosis can occur at any point along the path of the radiation and may be confused with persistent cancer. Similarly, mucosal ulcers can be produced in the bladder, vagina or rectum. These radiation ulcers are ischemic from the reduction in tissue vascularity produced by the radiation and are subject to necrosis by injudicious biopsies. The ability of these fibrotic tissues to form granulation tissue or to exhibit normal wound healing is permanently impaired. Consequently, the placement of surgical incision, and particularly of angulated surgical incisions, through either an entry or an exit port may be followed by delay or failure of wound healing (Spratt, 1962).

Patients with carcinoma of the bladder should have similar bi-manual pelvic examinations as well as cystoscopy. Particular attention is directed toward any palpable evidence of extension outside the bladder.

Most patients with invasive cancer of the bladder have a urinary tract infection. The infected cases are at risk to develop bacteremia spontaneously or after palpatory examination or other surgical manip-ulations. Consequently, these patients should be placed on broad-spectrum or bacteria-specific antibiotics before, during and after pel-vic examination and after cystoscopy. They are also prone to urinary bleeding and the filling of the bladder with clots. This makes accurate examination by cystoscopy difficult and compounds the risk of bac-teremia.

Histological confirmation of the presence of pelvic neoplasm is obtained by standard biopsy techniques in all cases. One exception to this rule is progressive radiation necrosis with fistula formation. Progression of this situation may necessitate a definitive surgical operation in the absence of histologically proven persistent cancer.

Cancers of any pelvic organ can, in rare instances, be localized to the pelvic viscera but by local growth may have invaded the muscu-loskeletal pelvis. Conversely, tumors of the musculoskeletal pelvis may invade the pelvic viscera. In either instance, a combination of vis-ceral exenteration and hemipelvectomy or translumbar amputation may be curative in carefully selected cases. Brunschwig reported 3 per cent of his exenterations required simultaneous resection of the bony pelvis. Among these were combination exenterations and hemi-pelvectomies for cancer arising in the cervix uteri. Of these, one pa-tient survived 12 years.

RADIATION NECROSIS

The only acceptable indication for pelvic exenteration in the ab-sence of histologically proven persistent cancer is radiation necrosis. The basic healing properties of tissues change after radiation (Spratt, 1962). Every photon traversing living tissue produces an ionized tract potentially damaging to all living cells on a random hit basis. The degree of damage varies with the time-dose factors, type of radiation, physical distribution of the radiation and tissue sensitivity. The toler-ance of cells varies, but vascular endothelium is one of the more radiosensitive tissues. As a result of the vascular injury, all irradiated tissues have a reduced vascularity. Capillaries in the irradiated tissue have a deficient capacity for budding which is necessary to form granulation tissue. The devascularized tissue is subject to progressive necrosis, sometimes developing spontaneously but often precipitated and always aggravated by infection or mechanical trauma. As a result of these changes, operative wounds within irradiated tissue heal more slowly and sometimes not at all. Necrosis may be progressive if started in this devascularized tissue by either trauma or infection.

As sequelae, the pelvic surgeon may find multiple organ fistulas, mucosal ulcers of pelvic viscera, extensive infection and pelvic pain requiring excisional therapy.

This radionecrotic process can result in the development of extensive visceral necrosis with a variety of fistulas — rectovaginal, vesicovaginal, ureterovaginal, enterovaginal and various other combinations. These fistulas may develop in the absence of persistent cancer. Prodromal causes include extensive cancers that necrose under treatment, ill-planned radiation therapy with poor dosage distribution, oversensitive response to the radiation therapy sometimes aggravated by the presence of infection, and injudicious biopsies. Once started, the necrosis often progresses throughout the field of radiation, and the end result is equivalent to a cloaca. Hence, the term cloacal syndrome refers to one of the most severe problems associated with advanced pelvic cancer.

Regardless of the prodromal cause, existence of this problem necessitates certain observations and decisions based on previous experience. First, it is desirable, but not necessary, to ascertain the presence or absence of residual cancer in the pelvis before starting any attempt at surgical management. Obtaining the diagnosis and evaluation necessitates a very careful pelvic examination under general anesthesia with the performance of selected biopsies of the margins of the fistulas and needle biopsies of nodular adnexal infiltrations. In the presence of recrudescent cancer, the fixation to the bony pelvis must be ascertained. Evaluation is effected by bimanual examination.

If the suspected cancerous fixation is movable even slightly, then a plane for dissection usually exists between the parietal layer of pelvic fascia and the pelvic parieties, and resection may be possible.

However, the presence of fistula formation is associated with much more intense adnexal scarring and infection than is present in the absence of fistulas and infection. When this occurs, colostomy and ileal bladder may be indicated initially. Diversionary operations to bypass the fistulas and the treatment of associated infections are a necessary prelude to the performance of exenterative surgery. The diversionary surgery may be the only treatment that is necessary or desirable in the absence of recurrent cancer. It may be the only form of palliation available in the presence of unresectable local cancer.

Pelves with fistulas in the absence of recurrent cancer have generally experienced a more intense radiational effect, and resective surgery is both more difficult and more frequently associated with major postoperative complications.

The surgical mortality rate after exenterations for this problem has been very high in the hands of all reporting authors (Sugg, Deckers, 1971; Ketcham, 1970). The irradiated pelvic wall is rigid and will not collapse, and the tissues lining the rigid cavity have lost their capacity to form granulation tissue. Thus, there is poor wound healing. Events resulting from this abnormality include infection, further intestinal fistulas, necrosis of the iliac vessels and loss of fluid and proteins through the large wound. The rate of caloric loss through the wound has never been measured.

When this syndrome develops, a permanent ileoneocystostomy and a descending end colostomy should be performed to divert completely the urine and fecal streams. The intestinal stomata must be placed in normal, nonirradiated skin, and similarly, the intestine used for this purpose must have received the least radiation. To appreciate the extent of irradiated skin, the surgeon must consult the radiotherapist before the operation to ascertain the site of radiation entry and exit ports and the approximate dosage received in the ports. Placement of intestinal stomata in or adjacent to these ports is associated

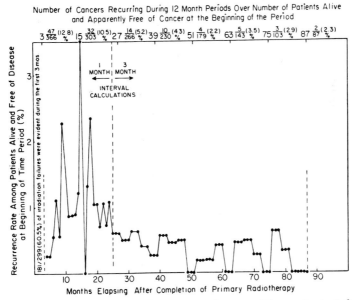

Figure 4–1   The interval rate of recurrence of cancer of the cervix uteri after radiotherapy, calculated by dividing the number of patients alive and "free of disease" at the beginning of a given time interval into the number of cancers that recurred during the ensuing interval. (From Gary, R. K., Sala, J. M., and Spratt, J. S., Jr.: The detection and treatment of postirradiationally recidivated cancers of the cervix uteri. Radiology, 83:208, 1964.)

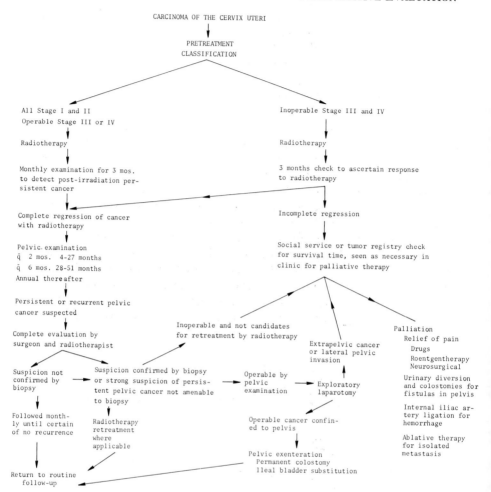

CARCINOMA OF THE CERVIX UTERI

PRETREATMENT
CLASSIFICATION

All Stage I and II
Operable Stage III or IV

Inoperable Stage III and IV

Radiotherapy

Radiotherapy

Monthly examination for 3 mos.
to detect post-irradiation persistent cancer

3 months check to ascertain response
to radiotherapy

Complete regression of cancer
with radiotherapy

Incomplete regression

Pelvic examination
q̄ 2 mos. 4-27 months
q̄ 6 mos. 28-51 months
Annual thereafter

Social service or tumor registry check
for survival time, seen as necessary in
clinic for palliative therapy

Persistent or recurrent pelvic
cancer suspected

Complete evaluation by
surgeon and radiotherapist

Inoperable and not candidates
for retreatment by radiotherapy

Palliation
   Relief of pain
      Drugs
      Roentgentherapy
      Neurosurgical

Extrapelvic cancer
or lateral pelvic
invasion

Suspicion not
confirmed by
biopsy

Suspicion confirmed by biopsy
or strong suspicion of persistent pelvic cancer not amenable
to biopsy

Operable by
pelvic
examination

Exploratory
laparotomy

Urinary diversion
and colostomies for
fistulas in pelvis

Followed month-
ly until certain
of no recurrence

Radiotherapy
retreatment
where
applicable

Operable cancer confin-
ed to pelvis

Internal iliac ar-
tery ligation for
hemorrhage

Ablative therapy
for isolated
metastasis

Pelvic exenteration
Permanent colostomy
Ileal bladder substitution

Return to routine
follow-up

Figure 4–2 Recommended follow-up plan based on the study of the interval recurrence rate and the efficacy of retreatment of persistent or recurrent carcinomas of the cervix uteri. (From Gary, R. K., Sala, J. M., and Spratt, J. S., Jr.: The detection and treatment of postirradiationally recidivated cancers of the cervix uteri. Radiology, 83:208, 1964.)

with frequent necrosis and intractable skin irritation. The stomata are ideally placed through nonirradiated abdominal walls as far away as possible from the irradiated skin and bony prominences. Location of stomata are thus affected by very important principles in these cases which have precedence over other routines. The sites for stomata must be selected and marked before abdominal landmarks are covered by sterile drapes. The intestine can be brought through these marked sites at appropriate phases of the operative procedure, but the proper locations are difficult to determine in a draped patient if the properly selected sites have not been marked before draping.

Among 16 pelvic exenterations performed for persistent radiational injury, five patients died postoperatively. Four of these five patients were operated upon for necrosis of the irradiated pelvic tissue that continued to progress after urinary and fecal diversion (Sugg).

When radiation therapy fails to control the cancer of the cervix uteri, recurrent neoplasm is diagnosed with a definable temporal pattern, as shown in Figure 4–1. On the basis of this pattern, a schedule for follow-up examination has been developed that gives a 2 per cent recurrence rate per follow-up examination after primary radiotherapy of cancers of the cervix uteri (Fig. 4–2). Following this schedule should permit the diagnosis of cancers locally recurrent in the pelvis after primary treatment while the recurrent cancer may still be amenable to control by pelvic exenteration.

EARLY INDICATIONS FOR PELVIC EXENTERATION

A system for identifying and following patients most at risk to develop recrudescent pelvic neoplasms amenable to control by exenterative surgery can be helpful in discovering pelvic cancers before they become unresectable.

At practically every anatomical site neoplasms can occur that do not metastasize outside the pelvis and that are ultimately responsible for the demise of the patient because of local persistence and progression. These cancers are identifiable on the basis of clinical and pathological information acquired at a previous time of treatment. The most frequent sites of recurrent cancers amenable to further curative therapy are the cervix uteri and rectum. Consequently, the follow-up system requisite to identify these cases is separately considered.

To date, the two most helpful parameters in the case of the cervix uteri have been the stage of the cancer before radiation therapy and the appearance of the ureters as seen on intravenous pyelography (Gary, Waggoner).

In the following cancer patients who have had pelvic cancer treated primarily by radiation therapy or surgery, the most important procedures are direct inspection and palpation by an experienced observer. Ideally, each examination should be performed by the same observer who will record and compare his successive findings in search for change. No single method of examination is absolute. The site of recurrence and signs most frequently associated with recurrent cancer of the cervix uteri after radiotherapy are given in Figure 4–3.

The material on which conclusions are based includes data from the treatment of 554 consecutive patients seen at the EFSCH between 1950 and 1959 with previously untreated cancer of the cervix uteri.

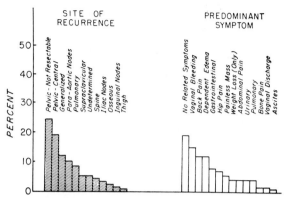

Figure 4-3 Principal sites of recurrence and predominant symptoms manifested by postirradiationally recidivated cancer of the cervix uteri. (From Gary, R. K., Sala, J. M., and Spratt, J. S., Jr.: The detection and treatment of postirradiationally recidivated cancers of the cervix uteri. Radiology, *83*:208, 1964.)

Cases were staged according to the 1950 League of Nations criteria. Cystoscopic and sigmoidoscopic examinations, intravenous pyelography and thoracic roentgenography were performed routinely on each patient. All of the cancers in this series were treated primarily by radiotherapy. The total experience is given in Table 4–1. The high treatment failure rate by radiation therapy for both stage III and stage IV cancers and the frequency of persistence and recurrence with more advanced stages of the neoplasms are clearly in evidence. This high treatment failure rate for advanced stage cancers managed initially by radiation therapy may indicate a need for earlier consideration of exenteration for cancers of the cervix uteri apparently restricted to the pelvis but not controllable by radiation therapy, as suggested by Deckers (1972). Experience in the management of advanced cancers that persist or recur after radiation therapy has confirmed that some of these neoplasms are advanced local cancers without the propensity to metastasize even to the regional lymph nodes. For these cases, primary exenterative resection in the absence of previous radiation would enhance the chances for primary wound healing without numerous secondary complications associated with extensive surgery in an irradiated pelvis.

When recurrent cancer is suspected, biopsy is necessary to prove the presence of cancer. Exposed areas can be biopsied directly with appropriate biopsy forceps. When nodularity or suspicious thickening of paracervical ligaments is detected, these can be biopsied transvaginally with a Franklin needle or Vim-Silverman needle. Sequential observation by the same examiner is important in identifying the areas that require biopsy. Any abnormal physical finding that undergoes progressive advancement on successive observations must be considered as being caused by residual cancer until proved otherwise by reversal or the progressive abnormality.

Still seen from time to time are ulcers of the bladder, vagina or rectum produced by radiotherapy. These are characterized by fairly sharp mucosal margins and a white or gray relatively avascular scar in the base of the ulcer and can often be differentiated from cancer by inspection. Unnecessary biopsy of these ulcers can accelerate the radionecrotic process causing the ulcer.

As long as radiation therapy is used as primary treatment, it is nec-

Table 4-1   Survival of Patients Treated Primarily by Roentgen Therapy at the Ellis Fischel State Cancer Hospital from 1950 to 1959[*]

	Median Age	No. of Patients	Period (yrs.)	Accumulative Survival (%)	Expected Survival (%)[**]	Accumulative Survival Adjusted for Natural Mortality (%)[†]
Stage I[‡]	45	88(15.9%)	3	85.17	98.9	86.1
			5	82.83	98.0	84.5
			7	75.81	96.3	78.7
Stage II[‡]	51	113(20.4%)	3	62.80	98.1	64.0
			5	51.10	96.6	52.9
			7	50.19	94.9	52.9
Stage III[‡]	55	272(49.1%)	3	47.39	97.4	48.7
			5	42.98	95.3	45.1
			7	40.24	92.9	43.3
Stage IV[‡]	57	81(14.6%)	3	16.03	96.9	16.5
			5	14.80	94.5	15.7
			7	11.10	91.6	12.1
All stages[‡]	54	554(100%)	3	50.62	97.6	51.9
			5	45.70	95.4	47.9
			7	39.07	93.2	41.9
Untreated recurrences[§]	51	272(49.1%)	3	1.83	98.1	1.86
			5	1.09	96.6	1.13
			7	0.36	94.9	0.38
Treated recurrences[§,§§]	47	27(4.9%)	3	53.89	98.7	54.6
			5	53.89	97.6	55.2
			7	53.89	96.3	56.0

[*]From Gary, R. K., Sala, J. M., and Spratt, J. S., Jr.: The detection and treatment of post-irradiationally recidivated cancers of the cervix uteri. Radiology, 83:208, 1964.

[**]Missouri State Life Tables for white females, 1949–1951. Life Tables for 1949–1951; Vol. 41, No. 4. Life Tables for Geographic Divisions of the United States (Missouri). U.S. Department of Health, Education and Welfare, National Office of Vital Statistics, Special Reports. Washington D.C., U.S. Government Printing Office, 1956.

[†]Finney, p. 88, Abbott's formula. (Finney, D. J.: Probit Analysis, A Statistical Treatment of the Sigmoid Response Curve. 2nd ed. London, Cambridge University Press, 1962.)

[‡]Survival measured from time of first admission for cervical cancer.

[§]Survival measured from time recurrence or persistence diagnosed.

[§§]Implies treatment of central pelvic recurrence or persistence by pelvic exenteration or additional roentgen therapy. These women were obviously good risk patients, since none have died of other causes if their cancers were effectively controlled by retreatment.

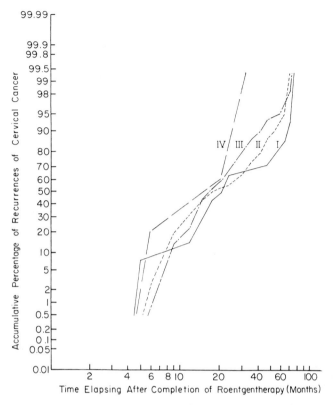

Figure 4-4 Accumulative percentage of cancers of the cervix uteri recurring after roentgen therapy, according to pretreatment stage. Calculations begin with the end of the third post-treatment month. (From Gary, R. K., Sala, J. M., and Spratt, J. S., Jr.: The detection and treatment of postirradiationally recidivated cancers of the cervix uteri. Radiology, 83:208, 1964.)

essary to appreciate the temporal patterns of persistence and recurrence in order to design a follow-up system that will permit the timely diagnosis of still resectable neoplasm. The temporal skew of persistence and recurrence through the ninetieth post-treatment month is given in Figure 4–4. This temporal pattern was affected only slightly by the pretreatment stage of the neoplasm. If the neoplasm regressed after the primary course of radiation therapy, 50 per cent of the recurrence became evident by the twentieth post-treatment month. By the use of an early, rather nonsystematic, follow-up system, the principal sites of recurrence and predominant symptoms manifested by the recidivous cancer are given in Figure 4–3. Based on the analysis of the data contained in this study, a critical path for the follow-up of carcinoma of the cervix uteri is shown in Figure 4–2. The potential and actual results of retreatment after radiotherapeutic failure are shown in Table 4–2. Long-term survivors occasionally develop additional primary pelvic cancers that must be managed by pelvic exenteration (Ketcham, 1970).

The intravenous pyelogram can be extremely helpful in identifying patients at greater risk to develop recurrent carcinoma of the cer-

Table 4–2 Frequency, Method and Result of Retreating 299 Cancers of the Cervix Uteri Persistent or Recurrent After Radiotherapy*

	LEAGUE OF NATIONS STAGE				
	I	II	III	IV	TOTALS
Group					
Number of cancers of the cervix uteri receiving initial radiotherapy at the Ellis Fischel State Cancer Hospital, 1950–1959	88	113	272	81	554
I. Number of cancers not controlled by radiotherapy	20	50	156	73	299
A. Persistent cancers	2(10%)	12(24%)	95(61%)	67(92%)	176(58.7%)
B. Recurrent cancers	18(90%)	38(76%)	59(38%)	6(8%)	121(40.7%)
C. Not known whether persistent or recurrent	0	0	2	0	2
II. Cancer thought localized to central pelvis by pelvic examination when persistence or recurrence discovered	9	17	35	4	65
A. Cancer electively retreated radiologically	2	3	2	0	7
1. Cancer not controlled	0	0	2	0	2
2. Cancer controlled	2	3	0	0	5
B. Abdominal exploration for pelvic exenteration	7	13	30	4	54
1. Inoperable by abdominal exploration	3	9	19	3	34
2. Exenteration performed, cancer not controlled**	2	4	5	0	11
3. Exenteration performed, cancer controlled	2	0	6	1	9
III. Clinically inoperable when recurrence or persistence discovered	11	33	121	69	234
A. Locally advanced	3	20	49	4	76
B. Metastases present	8	8	48	21	85
C. Nature of recurrence not determined†	0	5	24	44	73

*From Gary, R. K., Sala, J. M., and Spratt, J. S., Jr.: The detection and treatment of post-irradiationally recidivated cancers of the cervix uteri. Radiology, 83:208, 1964.
**Includes six postoperative deaths.
†Died in first several months after treatment—not seen in clinic after treatment.

vix uteri after radiation therapy that may require pelvic exenteration to control the uncured cancer. Waggoner and Spratt reviewed the prognostic significance of intravenous pyelographic observations in 945 cases of carcinoma of the cervix uteri treated primarily by radiation therapy:

A tumor recurrence rate of 93.5 per cent followed irradiation therapy when pretreatment abnormal intravenous pyelogram changes were present. This rate was essentially the same regardless of clinical stage of disease. Persistence or development of obstructive pelvic ureteropathy after irradiation was associated in follow-up with tumor recurrence. The only exceptions were those cases developing vesicovaginal fistulas. Ureteropathy attributable to irradiation effect was rare, even in the presence of severe postirradiation morbidity of pelvic viscera. Only four cases were so classified in this group. Abnormal intravenous pyelogram changes developing with post-therapy tumor recurrence were also associated with reduced tumor control by retreatment. Operative pelvic exenteration produced a 19 per cent control in a small group of such cases.

REFERENCES

Brunschwig, A., and Barber, H. R. K.: Pelvic exenteration combined with resection of segments of bony pelvis. Surgery, 65:417, 1969.

Cunningham, C. J., Watson, F. R., Spratt, J. S., Jr., and Hahn, R. C.: Behavioral sciences and cancer, a review. Mo. Med., 68:896, 1971.

Deckers, P. J., Ketcham, A. S., Sugarbaker, E. V., Hoye, R. C., and Thomas, L. B.: Pelvic exenteration for primary carcinoma of the uterine cervix. Obstet. Gynecol., 37:647, 1971.

Deckers, P. J., Sugarbaker, E. V., Pilch, Y. H., and Ketcham, A. S.: Pelvic exenteration for late second cancers of the uterine cervix after earlier irradiation. Ann. Surg., 175:48, 1972.

Gary, R. K., Sala, J. M., and Spratt, J. S., Jr.: The detection and treatment of postirradiationally recidivated cancers of the cervix uteri. Radiology, 83:208, 1964.

Ketcham, A. S., Deckers, P. J., Sugarbaker, E. V., Hoye, R. C., Thomas, L. B., and Smith, R. R.: Pelvic exenteration for carcinoma of the uterine cervix, a 15-year experience. Cancer, 26:513, 1970.

Ketcham, A. S., Harrah, J. D., Deckers, P. J., Rabson, A. S., and Chretien, P. B.: Scalene fat pad biopsy as a determinant in the success of therapy of carcinoma of the cervix. (In press.)

Moyer, C. A.: The assessment of operative risk. In Moyer, C. A., and others: Surgery, Principles and Practices. 3rd ed. Philadelphia, J. B. Lippincott Co., 1965.

Spratt, J. S., Jr., and Sala, J. M.: The healing of wounds within irradiated tissue. Mo. Med., 59:409, 1962.

Spratt, J. S., Jr., Shieber, W., and Dillard, B. M.: Anatomy and Surgical Technique of Groin Dissection. Saint Louis, The C. V. Mosby Co., 1965.

Sugg, W. L., Lawler, W. H., Ackerman, L. V., and Butcher, H. R., Jr.: Operative therapy for severe irradiational injury in the enteral and urinary tracts. Ann. Surg., 157:62, 1963.

Waggoner, C. M., and Spratt, J. S., Jr.: Prognostic significance of radiographic ureteropathy before and after irradiation therapy for carcinoma of the cervix uteri. Am. J. Obstet. Gynecol., 105:1197, 1969.

Chapter Five

PREOPERATIVE
MANAGEMENT

This section emphasizes the technical aspects of preoperative preparation. However, the listing of the technical preparative steps is best preceded by consideration of social, psychological and economic factors. Patients undergoing exenterative surgery are faced with no alternative if they wish to live because they have problems that are otherwise lethal. They will end up with considerably altered bodily functions, permanent intestinal stomata and the loss of sexual function. These are all psychologically stressful conditions that only the mentally sound and those with a stronger than average will to live can tolerate. No controlled studies exist on the selection of those with mental stamina necessary, but a growing literature deals with the complex and unusual aberrations that such stresses can produce (Cunningham).

PSYCHOLOGICAL AND SOCIAL PREPARATION

No absolute guidelines exist for avoiding undue psychological trauma, and the authors can only offer their attitude, which is a compromise between the lethality of the medical problems requiring the exenteration, the medicolegal necessity for informed consent and the need for patient and family understanding, cooperation and participation during the preoperative, postoperative and rehabilitative processes. First, there are certain things the patient and family have to know. Second, there are additional things they will wish to know.

79

Third, the patient must be motivated to participate in the recuperative phases. Fourth, the most stressful psychological trauma seems to come from uncertainty and anxiety which can only be alleviated by informative and supportive communication among the patient, the physician and *all* other persons interacting with the patient. The patient's entire social web before and after the operation should serve a positive supportive role in his best interest.

The diagnosis of cancer is a shock to any person and almost invariably has a disruptive effect on the personality because many people still believe all cancer to be incurable (Shands et al., Currier). Actually it is probably the most curable of all chronic diseases. Even when cure is not possible, long periods of symptom-free survival can be obtained. Physicians are also able to speak with greater assurance about the probable outcome of treatment as well-monitored clinical data continue to accumulate. At one time in the past patients with advanced cancer would have been considered incurable. With proper selection and care they often have a good chance for quality survival. At least one physician has three of these patients who are now more than 20 years past their exenteration (Healey). Properly transmitted, this information could alleviate much of the initial stress on patient and family.

Many patients' fear of cancer also lies in their fear of the problems surrounding changes produced by treatment. Pelvic exenteration requires major surgery. The changes in the form and function of several body organs are extensive and occur in a matter of hours. The patient's attitude toward surgery itself and the organs it affects and the attitude of those around him may determine the final outcome of the procedure.

Consideration of the patient's psychological health begins with his selection for pelvic exenteration. This operation should not be done just because the patient has not responded to other treatment and is therefore going to die. The ultimate objective is to place him back in his home, happy in his existence and hopefully in gainful employment. The individual's psyche and ability to handle problems must be considered. "There is no more stressful phenomenon in the world than to have to go through a pelvic exenteration procedure... they've got to be able to get through that and after that, be able to have enough psychiatric stability to be able to make the adjustment over into their physiological state, which is profound" (Healey).

The patient's adaptation to this procedure begins with the discovery that something is wrong with his health, progresses for better or worse during the preoperative period, culminates with surgery, evolves during the postoperative and convalescent stages toward the final resolution and depends a great deal on the professional help he receives during the entire time (Sutherland, 1952). The problems he faces are not those normally found in everyday life, nor are they problems for which he has a great deal of preparation.

Any reasonable predication of the patient's reaction to the loss of function he will undergo can only be made by knowing the value system and vulnerable areas of that particular patient (Hollender). Improved psychological histories for each patient would be of benefit (Payne et al.). Specialized personnel can be employed to discover the specific, indirect and/or symbolic effect of the loss on the patient in order to meet his needs more effectively (Hollender). At least one author believes cancers at certain sites will bring about certain psychological processes or aberrations (Fras et al.). Some research has been done on site-specific problems encountered by pelvic exenteration patients (Dyk et al., Knorr, Healey), but the effect of the patient's psychological make-up and emotional support from those around him on his ability to readjust needs further systematic study in a larger context. The patient's adaptation is by no means static and is not at any time independent of concurrent life situations (Sutherland, 1952).

Psychological problems are probably most dramatic during the preoperative period while the patient is still hospitalized. He is alone and free to reflect on his condition, imagining all sorts of outcomes which may or may not be realistic (Sutherland, 1967). There is the possibility of recurrence, postoperative complications or operative death. But the fear of mutilation is probably the worst. Because of his self-image, a person may fear this more than death (Aronson). What the patient hears or is told at this stage could very well have a significant effect on his overall adaptation.

The patient must be prepared to accept his altered condition before treatment begins (Sutherland, 1967; Adsett; Healey; Callaway; Gardner; Dietz). However, care should be taken when communicating with the patient about his treatment course. For instance, "radical surgery" suggests a destructive procedure and is difficult to associate with good health. "Definitive surgery" is a less traumatic term (Sutherland, 1967). The word "tumor" could be substituted for the word "cancer" in some cases. The problem of communication with the cancer patient needs in-depth study and continual evaluation and research (Edwards). There is a strong indication that a means of open communication is needed for the patient and his family to express their feelings about cancer on an individual basis (Baker et al., Abrams, Knapp, Waxenberg, Klagsburn). How patterns of communication change during the course of the disease is not yet known, but it is reasonable to suspect that cancer patients' communications cannot be interpreted in the same way as those of other patients (Abrams).

Closely associated with communication is the attitude displayed by the professionals. "Kindness, acceptance, and support, especially from professional persons have been proved over and over again to be of great significance to the patient" (Sutherland, 1952). The physician assumes the responsibility for the guidance, execution and final assessment of the treatment course. The nurse bears a greater burden, since she may be the only member of the medical team who is in sustained contact with the patient. In this respect she is the center of attention (Aronson). The social worker's training in meeting people's needs and in helping them to solve practical problems makes her a valuable ally in the struggle to resume normal functioning (Sutherland, 1952). The role of other medical and paramedical personnel in the total care of cancer patients is not clearly known. Even the maid who cleans the patient's room during the most stressful parasurgical periods may provide needed and beneficial support through her attitude and actions as perceived by the patient. Evaluation of the behavioral pattern of these individuals must be made in order to determine the pattern of greatest benefit to the patient.

The patient's response to altered bodily function is critically important to his welfare and rehabilitation. The notion that mutilation is a form of punishment for sin is common. His feelings of guilt can cause him to make heroic attempts to hide his distress from others (Barckley). Few people are prepared to be heroes by themselves and would be able to adjust better to their circumstances with professional help. The patient may perceive extensive surgical alteration as a serious injury which makes him too feeble and frail to resume normal functioning. One report quotes a patient as saying, "I have lost confidence in my body" (Sutherland, 1952). Depression and invalidism need adequate attention when they first appear, or the situation may become permanent.

Depression accompanied by dependence is to be expected in the majority of patients but should only be temporary. This normally precedes real progress, and its duration depends on the amount and kind of help he receives. In many cases it is simply enough to know that help is available. This fills the patient's need for security, and he may rely on it only occasionally, if at all (Sutherland, 1952).

Often regression persists because patients are left to rely totally on themselves or on the well-meant but inappropriate help of their families and friends. There is a lack of outside help for the patient who needs to talk to someone not as emotionally involved as these people are (Baker et al.). The surgeon's evaluation of the family situation seems of paramount importance, since the patient's adjustment in convalescence is closely related. The family can and does play an important supportive role (Norris; Bozeman et al.; Orbach et al.; Currier; Sutherland, 1967; Healey; Gardner; Knorr; Bouchard). Mediation by the health team in specific problem areas may provide insights to help the patient and his family reach a quicker and easier adjustment.

The patient's use of denial before or immediately after surgery is an important defense mechanism which reduces depression and anxiety too difficult for him to manage. It is not as useful after the illness and then may be detrimental (Knorr).

Other emotional reactions include hostility, hypochondria, counterphobia, obsession-compulsion and acute schizophrenia. All of these reactions usually occur together or in a series rather than separately (Adsett). Although the threat of suicide is more verbal than actual, the possibility exists in almost every case (Kline et al.). The recognition and proper management of these reactions require professional guidance and skills not formally given to the medical personnel who generally come in contact with the cancer patient. The necessary guidance may need to come from a psychiatrist, a psychologist, a social worker, a minister or other individuals with training in psychology, psychiatry or both. They should interact with the clinical team through consultation, collaboration, research and education. Rehabilitation requires careful consideration by all health team members, but the systematic study of the problems peculiar to exenteration have been surprisingly sparse (Baker et al., McGann, Abrams, Oken, Healey, Gardner, LaDue, Rothenberg).

The duration of psychological and social problems following discharge depends on the environment to which the patient is returned. The patient's physical disabilities are often compounded by fears of rejection. He must cope with the doubts of his employer and the community as well as his own. Frequently, agencies are ready to meet patient and family needs, but they are unaware of the patient, and he is often unaware of them. Or the reverse may be true. Some vocational counselors are not yet psychologically adjusted to accept cancer patients for retraining. In addition, they are rated on the number of closed cases they obtain and feel cancer cases could not be closed as readily as other types (Healey). The increased survival rate for cancer means a consequent increase in financial drain on the families affected and a necessary concern with the quality of the cancer patient's survival. Positive planning and understanding in the community is essential for total rehabilitation (Healey).

PREOPERATIVE CLINICAL EVALUATION

The preoperative studies should document the condition of the patient with reference to anemia, presence of sepsis (particularly of the urinary tract) and the existence of partial colonic or ureteral obstruction. The studies should also identify various medical problems requiring preoperative correction. For example, the patient with chronic lung disease may significantly benefit from a few days of preoperative therapy. (The same general aspects of pre- and postoperative care discussed in the American College of Surgeons book on the subject apply to patients who are to undergo exenterative pelvic surgery.)

The preoperative correction of anemia is achieved in most patients by the use of packed red blood cells to avoid excessive expansion of the blood volume and reduce the incidence of reactions to plasma proteins and possible transmission of serum hepatitis. A hemoglobin concentration of 10 gm. per 100 ml. is the minimum preoperative level.

If urinalysis shows bacilluria, proper cultures and antibiotic sensitivity studies should be performed. Specific antibiotic therapy should be given before, during and after surgery in patients with urinary tract infections. In the occasional patient not responding to specific therapy whose urinary tract infection seems progressive, the ileal bladder construction should precede exenteration by several weeks. The presence of obstructive uropathy or the presence of intravesical neoplasm may require the performance of an ileal bladder as a necessary prelude to the control of sepsis. The tolerance of the patient to subsequent exenteration is enhanced by the control of sepsis and azotemia. Failure to control or suppress urinary tract infection before performing the actual exenteration may result in septicemia and lethal septic complications. Ordinarily infection cannot be well controlled if it exists in the presence of partial or total urinary tract obstruction or in the presence of a fistula or foreign body such as a large bladder cancer.

Similarly, the presence of obstructive uropathy with an elevated BUN even in the absence of sepsis may make construction of a preliminary ileal bladder advisable. The preliminary ileal bladder is definitely indicated with an otherwise operable lesion for the patient in whom obstructive uropathy has produced an elevated BUN over 40 mg. per 100 ml. or in whom urinary tract sepsis cannot be improved on antibiotic therapy, as is frequently the case in the presence of urinary fistulas or ureteral obstruction with proximal infection.

Intestinal preparation in the days preceding the operation should be directed toward thorough mechanical cleansing of the intestine. In the absence of significant obstruction this can be well accomplished by minimum residue diet, cathartics and cleansing enemas of saline. Intestinal antibiotics are not routinely necessary in these patients. The presence or absence of partial colonic or rectal obstruction produced by cancer is the major determinant in selecting the method and duration of the preoperative preparation.

When partial intestinal obstruction exists cathartics may be contraindicated. In these cases preparation is necessarily limited to a minimum residue diet and daily small saline enemas until the proximal colon is mechanically clean. Confirmation of adequate cleansing after the enemas return clear can be secured by a roentgen examination of the abdomen that shows no retained feces. This cleansing process may take days of cautious effort in patients having a great deal of feces or barium entrapped proximal to the point of partial obstruction. A diverting colostomy is necessary for a completely obstructed colon. When staged colostomy is indicated, an end sigmoid colostomy should be constructed whenever possible. The proximal end of the distal sigmoid colon is closed but is brought to the abdominal skin level as the abdominal incision is closed. Rarely, in the presence of rectal obstruction, the proximal end of the distal sigmoid is sutured to the abdominal skin as a mucus fistula. If cancer is present on the mucosal surface of the bypassed sigmoid or rectum, the chances of implantation metastases in the abdominal wound about a mucus fistula are enhanced.

The usual preoperative routine for pelvic exenteration is as follows:

Review changes in technique and instrumentation with operating room supervisor and anesthesiologist.

Schedule several days ahead of time to allow a minimum of six hours operating time.

Order whole blood for intraoperative and postoperative transfusions; a minimum of six units should be available and cross-matched before the patient is anesthesized. If the patient has one of the less frequent blood types, additional units should be requested preoperatively.

Operation day minus five days: start on a minimum residue diet with daily multivitamin preparation.

Operation day minus five days: 30 cc. castor oil.

Operation day minus three days: 30 cc. castor oil.

Operation day minus two days: weigh, repeat mm. Hg pressures, Hct, WBC, BUN, FBS, serum concentrations of Na, K, Cl, CO_2 and other laboratory studies indicated for the particular patient.

Operation day minus one day: saline enemas until clear.

Administer a broad-spectrum antibiotic preoperatively, during the performance of the operation and continue three to four days postoperatively in all patients.

The night before surgery a sound night's sleep insures a rested body for the difficult day of surgery. Surgery is physical work for the patient and rest is necessary. Consequently, no cathartics are given on the day or evening before surgery. The evening meal before surgery should consist of a nonresidue diet containing liquids and semisolids of an amount sufficient to satisfy the patient's hunger and insure that he is well hydrated. No food or water is to be ingested after midnight.

His last saline enemas should be given early in the evening. Mild sedation should be given by 8 P.M., and by 9 P.M. he should be left undisturbed for the rest of the night so he can sleep. Unless there are genuine indications, it is unnecessary to awaken him in the middle of the night to check his vital signs. They can be checked at 6 A.M. before he is given his preoperative medication. The preoperative medications are then given according to the preference of the anesthesiologist. At the time preoperative medications are given, elastic stockings extending to the knee should be applied. These are worn during surgery and during the postoperative period. They are discontinued after the patient is ambulating without assistance.

Every patient having a pelvic exenteration will require a nasogastric tube during the operation and for at least the first five postoperative days. If preoperative studies suggest the presence of partial intestinal obstruction or consistent intestinal air patterns indicative of air swallowing, the nasogastric tube should be inserted one to several days before surgery. The tube is kept on low Gomco suction for drainage of the stomach. A slightly distended stomach and intestine, containing a little air or fluid, are extremely helpful during the exenteration. As will be discussed later, packing of these intestines out of the pelvis is necessary for exposure. When the intestines are too distended, the necessary degree of packing may not be mechanically feasible and, if forced, can press upward on the diaphragm, restricting pulmonary exchange, and can possibly restrict inferior vena cava return by pressure or by angular occlusion of the hepatic veins with resultant hypotension.

To improve the patient's understanding of his specific surgical setting and his potential areas of participation, careful preoperative education is helpful. The educational brochure used for all surgical patients at the EFSCH-CRC is reproduced in Appendix 2 as an example.

REFERENCES

Abrams, R. D.: The patient with cancer—his changing pattern of communication. N. Engl. J. Med., 274:317, 1966.

Abrams, R. D.: Social casework with cancer patients. Soc. Casework, 32:425, 1951.

Adsett, C. A.: Emotional reactions to disfigurement from cancer therapy. Can. Med. Assoc. J., 89:385, 1963.

Aronson, M. J.: Emotional aspects of nursing the cancer patient. Ment. Hyg., 42:267, 1958.

Baker, S. R., and Martin, L. R.: Paramedical needs of cancer patients. C.A., 14:59, 1964.

Barkcley, V.: What can I say to the cancer patient? Nurs. Outlook, 6:316, 1958.

Bouchard, R.: Psychological impact of cancer. In Bouchard, R.: Nursing Care of the Patient with Cancer. St. Louis, The C. V. Mosby Co., 1967.

Bozeman, M. F., Orbach, C. E., and Sutherland, A. M.: Psychological impact of cancer and its treatment. III. The adaptation of mothers to the threatened loss of their children through leukemia. Part I. Cancer, 8:1, 1955.

Callaway, E.: The psychological care of the cancer patient. J. Med. Assoc. Ga., *41*:502, 1952.

Cunningham, C. J., Watson, F. R., Spratt, J. S., Jr., and Hahn, R. C.: Behavioral sciences and cancer, a review. Mo. Med., *68*:896, 1971.

Currier, L. M.: The psychological impact of cancer on the cancer patient and his family. Rocky Mt. Med. J., *63*:43, 1966.

Dietz, J. H.: Rehabilitation of the cancer patient. Med. Clin. North Am., *53*:607, 1969.

Dyk, R. B., and Sutherland, A. M.: Adaptation of the spouse and other family members to the colostomy patient. Cancer, *9*:123, 1956.

Edwards, H. D.: Discussion on palliation in cancer. Proc. R. Soc. Med., *48*:35, 1955.

Fras, I., and Litin, E. M.: Comparison of psychiatric manifestations in carcinoma of the pancreas, retroperitoneal malignant lymphoma, and lymphoma in other locations. Psychosomatics, *8*:275, 1967.

Gardner, W. H.: Adjustment problems of laryngectomized women. Arch. Otolaryngol., *83*:57, 1966.

Healey, J. E., Jr. (ed.): Ecology of the Cancer Patient: Proceedings of Three Interdisciplinary Conferences on Rehabilitation of the Cancer Patient. Washington, D.C., Interdisciplinary Communications Associates, Inc., 1970.

Hollender, M. H.: The physician, the patient, and cancer. Ill. Med. J., *107*:20, 1955.

Kinney, J. M., Egdahl, R. H., and Zuidema, G. D.: Manual of Preoperative and Postoperative Care. 2nd ed. Philadelphia, W. B. Saunders Co., 1971.

Klagsburn, S. C.: Communications in the treatment of cancer. Am. J. Nurs., *71*:944–948, 1971.

Kline, N., and Sobin, J.: Psychological management of cancer patients. J.A.M.A., *146*:1547, 1951.

Knapp, M.: How do you feel about cancer? Nurs. Outlook, *2*:350, 1954.

Knorr, N. J.: A depressive syndrome following pelvic exenteration and ileostomy. Arch. Surg., *94*:258, 1967.

LaDue, J. S.: The management of terminal patients with inoperable cancer. J. Kans. Med. Soc., *54*:1, 1953.

McGann, L. M.: The cancer patient's needs: How can we meet them? J. Rehabil., *30*:19, 1964.

Norris, A. S.: Personality reactions to the diagnosis of cancer. J. Iowa Med. Soc., *57*:344, 1967.

Oken, D.: What to tell cancer patients. J.A.M.A., *175*:1120, 1961.

Orbach, C. E., Sutherland, A. M., and Bozeman, M. F.: Psychological impact of cancer and its treatment. III. The adaptation of mothers to the threatened loss of their children through leukemia: Part II. Cancer, *8*:20, 1955.

Payne, E. C., and Krant, M. J.: The psychological aspects of advanced cancer. J.A.M.A., *210*:1238, 1969.

Rothenberg, A.: Psychological problems in terminal cancer management. Cancer, *14*:1063, 1961.

Shands, H. C., Finesinger, J. E., Cobb, S., and Abrams, R. D.: Psychological mechanisms in patients with cancer. Cancer, *4*:1159, 1951.

Sutherland, A.: Psychological impact of cancer surgery. Public Health Rep., *67*:1139, 1952.

Sutherland, A. M.: Psychological observations in cancer patients. Int. Psychiat. Clin., *4*:75, 1967.

Waxenberg, S. E.: The importance of the communication of feelings about cancer. Ann. N.Y. Acad. Sci., *125*:1000, 1966.

Chapter Six

ANESTHESIA

The selection of anesthesia is largely the responsibility of the anesthesiologist. Pelvic exenterations have been performed under all types of general endotracheal anesthesia, and the type the anesthesia team is most familiar with for prolonged operations is probably the best. The factors that are unique to the operation include the need for the intraoperative blood and fluid replacement requisite to maintain a normotensive patient with an unrestricted urinary output. As a precautionary measure, central venous pressure should be monitored.

Two securely implanted 15 gauge needles or intravenous catheters are necessary for the administration of blood, fluids and drugs intraoperatively and the monitoring of central venous pressure. Because of the multiplicity of intravenous administrations, the potential incompatibility of drugs with other drugs, blood, components of fluid in which the drugs are administered and abnormal patient sensitivity must all be carefully monitored by the person in charge of intravenous therapy. A recent list of incompatible relationships is given in Table 6–1.

Table 6–1   Incompatibilities of Commonly Used Drugs for Intravenous Administration

AGENT	INCOMPATIBLE AGENTS
Antibiotics	
Amphotericin B*	Potassium penicillin G, tetracyclines
Cephalothin	Calcium chloride or calcium gluconate, erythromycin, polymyxin B, tetracyclines
Chloramphenicol (Chloromycetin)	B-complex vitamin preparations, hydrocortisone, polymyxin B, tetracyclines, vancomycin
Methicillin**	Tetracyclines
Nafcillin	B-complex vitamin preparations
Potassium penicillin G	Amphotericin B, metaraminol, phenylephrine, tetracyclines, vancomycin, ascorbic acid
Polymyxin B	Cephalothin, chloramphenicol, heparin, tetracyclines
Tetracyclines†	Amphotericin B, cephalothin, chloramphenicol, heparin, hydrocortisone, methicillin, potassium penicillin G, polymyxin B
Vancomycin	Chloramphenicol, heparin, hydrocortisone, potassium penicillin G
Pressors	
Ephedrine	Hydrocortisone
Epinephrine	Mephentermine
Mephentermine	Epinephrine
Meteraminol	Potassium penicillin G
Phenylephrine‡	Potassium penicillin G
Miscellaneous	
Aminophylline	Acidic solutions, B-complex vitamin preparations, barbiturates, calcium or magnesium salts, vancomycin
B-complex vitamin preparations	Aminophylline, chloramphenicol, hydrocortisone, nafcillin
Barbiturates and tranquilizers	Many drugs
Calcium chloride or calcium gluconate	Cephalothin, sodium bicarbonate, tetracyclines
Heparin	Tetracyclines, polymyxin B, vancomycin
Hydrocortisone	B-complex vitamin preparations, chloramphenicol, ephedrine, tetracyclines, vancomycin
Sodium bicarbonate	Calcium chloride or calcium gluconate, lactated Ringer's solution

*Specific instructions for reconstitution are provided by the manufacturer; the agent should always be administered alone.

**Physical stability or biological potency may change after reconstitution; the agent should be administered alone soon after it is diluted.

†The agent should not be mixed with solutions which contain calcium. Ringer's solution may be used as a diluent because the pH of that solution is acid.

‡Bisulfite is used as an antioxidant in commercial preparations of this agent; bisulfite slowly inactivates penicillin G.

Chapter Seven

OPERATIVE SETTING
AND EQUIPMENT

THE OPERATING ROOM

Requirements peculiar to exenterative pelvic operations include the need for adequate floor space. The room must accommodate instrument tables for both an abdominal and a perineal instrument set, an orthopedic table with abduction leg extensions, lights for simultaneous illumination of abdominal and perineal fields, space for abdominal and perineal surgical teams, anesthesia equipment and staff, two scrub nurses and two circulating nurses. We find that a room 20' by 20' is the minimum size which will accommodate all phases of the procedure.

SURGICAL INSTRUMENTS

The instruments necessary to perform exenterative surgery of the pelvis are listed in Table 7–1. Major contraindications to the performance of exenterations are the lack of proper instruments for exposure, dissection and hemostasis and the lack of familiarity with their usage.

Table 7–1 Surgical Instruments for Exenterative Pelvic Resections and Reconstruction °

Laparotomy Set of Instruments

No.	Item
1	#3 Bard-Parker surgery knife handle (Weck)
3	#4 Bard-Parker surgery knife handle (Weck)
1	#3L Bard-Parker deep surgery handle, straight (Weck)
1	#3LA Bard-Parker deep surgery handle, angled (Weck)
24	Crile hemostatic forceps, 6¼″, straight (Weck)
6	Crile hemostatic forceps, 6¼″, curved (Weck)
6	Mayo-Pean forceps, 8″ curved jaw (Weck)
12	Rochester-Pean forceps, 9″ curved jaw (Wester Brothers) W-15-321 lightweight model Pean made especially for Ellis Fischel
6	Mayo-Pean forceps, 10¼″ curved jaw (Weck)
6	Foerster sponge holding forceps, 9½″ straight serrated jaw (Weck)
24	Ochsner hemostats, 8″ straight (Weck)
4	Thoms-Allis tissue forceps, 8″, 6 × 7 teeth (Weck)
6	Babcock tissue forceps, 6¼″ (Weck)
2	Varco thoracic forceps, shallow curve, 7½″, box lock (Sklar)
1	Baby Sawtell hemostatic forceps, 7″ (right angle) (Baby Mixter) (Sklar)
3	Mayo-Hegar-Ochsner Diamond Jaw needle holder, 6″ (Snowden-Pencer)
3	Mayo-Hegar-Broad, Bulldog Jaw needle holder, 7″ (Weck)
3	Mayo-Hegar-Ochsner Diamond Jaw needle holder, 8″ (Snowden-Pencer)
1	Suture and wire cutting scissors 6″, straight, Wexteel (Weck)
2	Mixter suture scissors, 6″, straight, slender (Lawton)
2	Mayo dissecting scissors, 6¾″, lightweight, curved Wexteel (Weck)
2	Metzenbaum scissors, 7″, curved Wexteel (Weck)
3	Tissue forceps, 5½″, 2 × 3 teeth (Lawton)
2	Tissue forceps, 7″, 1 × 2 teeth (Lawton)
1	Tissue forceps, 10″, 1 × 2 teeth (Lawton)
3	Adson tissue forceps, 4¾″, 2 × 3 teeth (Lawton)
3	Dressing forceps, extra fine serrated tip, 5½″ (Lawton)
3	Dressing forceps, serrated tip, 7″ (Lawton)
2	Dressing forceps, serrated tip, 10″ (Lawton)
2	Dressing forceps, serrated tip, 12″ (Lawton)
1	Cushing vein and nerve retractor, 8″ (Weck)
2	Cushing vein and nerve retractor, 12″ (Weck)
2	Richardson retractor, regular handle, 2 × ¾″, blade 9½″ long (Weck)
2	Richardson retractor, regular handle, 1½″ × 1½″, blade 9½″ long (Weck)
2	Kelly abdominal retractor, 2½ × 2″ blade, 10″ long (Weck)
2	Kelly abdominal retractor, 3 × 2½″ blade, 10″ long (Weck)
2	Kelly abdominal retractor, 3½″ × 3″ blade, 9½″ long (Weck)
2	U.S. Army retractor (set of two), 8½″, with ⅝″ blade (Lawton)
1	Ochsner malleable retractor, 1″ wide, 13″ long (Weck)
1	Ochsner malleable retractor, 1½″ wide, 13″ long (Weck)
1	Ochsner malleable retractor, 2″ wide, 13″ long (Weck)
2	Deaver retractor, 1″ blade × 12″ (Lawton)
2	Deaver retractor, 2″ blade × 12″ (Lawton)
1	Deaver retractor, 3″ blade × 12″ (Lawton)
1	Harrington retractor, 2½″ blade, 12½″ long (Lawton)
2	Masson needle holder, thoracic, light model tungsten carbide jaws, 10½″ long (Lawton)
2	Masson needle holder, thoracic, 11½″ long tungsten carbide jaws (Sklar)
1	Nelson dissecting suture scissors, 9″ (Lawton)
1	Nelson dissecting suture scissors, 11″ (Lawton)

°All instruments referred to in this table are stainless steel unless otherwise noted.

Table 7–1 *continued on following page.*

Table 7–1   Surgical Instruments for Exenterative Pelvic Resections and Reconstruction (*Continued*)

1	Crafoord lobectomy scissors, 12″ curved blade (Weck)
1	Nelson lobectomy scissors, curved, thin, model 10 (Storz)
1	Metzenbaum scissors, operating, slim, curved, rounded blades, 9″ (Storz)
1	Willauer thoracic scissors, curved Wexteel, 10″ (Weck)
2	Mixter thoracic forceps, 9″, right angle (Lawton)
1	Mixter clamp forceps, angular jaw, 12″ (Weck)
4	Dennis anastomosis forceps, 9″ minimum trauma teeth (Lawton)
2	Doyen intestinal forceps, straight 9″ minimum trauma teeth (Lawton)
3	Yankauer suction tube, 9″ (Weck)
1	Poole abdominal suction tube, 8¾″ straight connection, 30 French (Weck)
1	Loré suction tubing and tip holding forceps (Weck)
8	Peers towel clamps, 5½″ (Lawton)
8	Backhaus towel clamp, 5¼″ (Weck)
1	Grieshaber Improved Balfour retractor unit, 10½″, with detachable lateral and center blade (United States Patent Number 2-693-795)
	3 pair wire lateral blades, 2½″, 3½″, 4½″
	1 center blade, 3″ wide, 3″ deep
	1 Purcell hysterectomy blade, 4″ wide, 3½″ deep
	1 center blade, 2½″ wide, 3½″ deep
	1 center blade, 3½″ wide, 4½″ deep (a specially made G5032 style) (Grieshaber)
1	Ruler, 6″ (V. Mueller)

Perineal Set of Instruments

2	#4 Bard-Parker surgery knife handle (Weck)
2	#4 Bard-Parker deep surgery knife handle (Weck)
1	Tissue forceps, 10″, 2 × 3 teeth (Weck)
2	Tissue forceps, 5½″, 2 × 3 teeth (Weck)
1	Dressing forceps, serrated tip, 10″ (Weck)
2	Volkman-Rake retractors, 8½″, sharp, 6 prongs (Lawton)
2	Ollier retractors, 8½″, 4 prongs, deep blunt (Lawton)
2	Mayo-Hegar needle holder, 7″, broad bulldog jaws (Weck)
2	Mayo dissecting scissors, 6¾″ curved, lightweight Wexteel (Weck)
2	Mixter suture scissors, 6″ straight, slender (Lawton)
1	Nelson dissecting suture scissors, straight 9″ (Lawton)
1	Nelson dissecting scissors, curved 9″ (Lawton)
2	Rochester-Pean forceps, 9″ curved (Wester Brothers)
	W-15-321 lightweight model Pean made especially for Ellis Fischel
2	Foerster sponge holding forceps, 9½″ straight (Weck)
4	Allis tissue forceps, 6″, 5 × 6 teeth (Weck)
6	Crile hemostatic forceps, 6¼″, straight (Weck)
1	Yankauer suction tube, 9″ (Weck)
24	Ochsner hemostats, 8″ straight (Weck)
6	Peers towel clamps, 5½″ nonpiercing (Lawton)

Special Instruments

2	Payr pylorus clamp, 8″, with 2½″ jaws (Weck)
1	Ford-Deaver retractor with Lamb wedge lock handle, 5″ deep, 2″ wide (Lawton)
1	Ford-Deaver retractor with Lamb wedge lock handle, 5″ deep, 3″ wide (Lawton)
1	Ford-Deaver retractor with Lamb wedge lock handle, 5″ deep, 4″ wide (Lawton)
Hemo-Clip Sets	
2	Samuels applying forceps, 8″ for medium clips (Weck)
2	Samuels applying forceps, 10½″ for medium clips (Weck)
2	Samuels applying forceps, 10½″ for large clips (Weck)
1	Wood removing forceps to remove a clip (Weck)
1	Hemo-Clip cartridge base (Weck)

Table 7–1 *continued on opposite page.*

Table 7–1 Surgical Instruments for Exenterative Pelvic Resections and Reconstruction (*Continued*)

	Hemo-Clip cartridges for above instruments
	Medium size (for 1.25- to 4.0-mm. vessels) 25 clips per cartridge, catalogue #523-100 (Weck)
	Large size (for 4- to 11-mm. vessels) 25 clips per cartridge, catalogue #523-170 (Weck)
1	Auto-Suture stapler TA-30 (United States Surgical Corporation)
1	Auto-Suture stapler GIA (United States Surgical Corporation)
	Auto-Suture disposable loading units (United States Surgical Corporation)
	TA-30 3.5 mm.
	TA-30 4.8 mm.
	GIA
2	Crile-Wood needle holders, 8″ Diamond Jaw (V. Mueller)
2	Potts-Smith tissue forceps, delicate, 9″ fine serrated tips (V. Mueller)
8	Viet-Harrington clamps, 12″ (colloquially called "sweep clamps"), catalogue #36L-350A (Lawton)
1	Nelson scissors, 14½″ curved, extra thin dissecting blades (Lawton) (may have to be special ordered, discontinued item)
2	Mayo needle holders, 14½″ Dura-Grip Jaw (Lawton)
2	Exenteration retractor, overall 31″, blade 8″ deep, designed by E. M. Bricker (Lawton)
1	Exenteration retractor, overall 25″, blade 9″ deep, designed by E. M. Bricker (Lawton)
6	Skillman hemostatic forceps, 5″ curved (Weck)
6	Skillman hemostatic forceps, 5″ straight (Weck)

Instruments Used on Ileal Segment
Special

	Auto-Suture stapler TA-30, 3.5 mm. loading unit (United States Surgical Corporation)
2	Crile-Wood needle holders, 8″ Diamond Jaw (V. Mueller)
2	Potts-Smith tissue forceps, delicate 9″ fine serrated tips (V. Mueller)
8	Skillman hemostatic forceps, 5″ (Weck)

Taken from regular laparotomy set

3–4	Dennis anastamosis forceps, 9″ minimum trauma teeth (Lawton)
1	Bard-Parker knife handle #3L (Weck)
1	Metzenbaum dissecting scissors, 7″, curved (Weck)
1	Mixter suture scissors, 6″, straight, slender (Lawton)
1	Nelson dissecting suture scissors, 9″, straight (Lawton)
6	Crile hemostatic forceps, 6¼″ (Weck)

Instruments Used on Colostomy and Ileal Segment to Suture Bowel to Skin°

1	Dressing forceps, extra fine serrated tip, 5½″ (Lawton)
1	Mayo-Hegar needle holder, 6″, Diamond Jaw (Snowden-Pencer)
1	Metzenbaum scissors, 7″, curved (Weck)
1	Mixter scissors suture, 6″, straight, slender (Lawton)

Cut-Down Tray Instruments and Supplies

1	Bard-Parker #3 knife handle (Weck)
1	Wutzler minor surgery scissors, 4¾″, curved Wexteel (Weck)
1	#10 Bard-Parker knife blade (Weck)
1	#15 Bard-Parker knife blade (Weck)
1	Mixter suture scissors, 6″, straight, slender (Lawton)
4	Halstead mosquito forceps, 5″, straight (Weck)

°These are from regular laparotomy set.

Table 7-1 *continued on following page.*

Table 7–1   Surgical Instruments for Exenterative Pelvic Resections
and Reconstruction   (*Continued*)

1	Crile hemostatic forceps, 6¼″, curved (Weck)
1	Crile-Wood needle holder, Diamond Jaw light pointed, 6″ (V. Mueller)
1	Adson tissue forceps, 4¾″, delicate 1 × 2 teeth plus serrations (V. Mueller)
1	Alm self-retaining retractor, large, 3″ (V. Mueller)
4	Backhaus towel clamp, 3″ (Lawton)
2	Medicine glasses – 1 ounce, 30 ml., glass (V. Mueller)
2	Allis intestinal forceps, 6″, 4 × 5 teeth (V. Mueller)
1	Becton-Dickinson Multifit Leur-Lok 3 ring control 5 cc. syringe (V. Mueller)
1	#25 Gauge needle, ⅝″ length hypodermic disposable monoject 200 (Sherwood Medical Industries)
1	#22 Gauge needle, 1½″ length hypodermic disposable monoject 200 (Sherwood Medical Industries)
4	Towels for draping incision, cotton huck-a-back
10	Sponges, 4 × 4 gauze (Johnson & Johnson)
1	Packet 4-0 silk with cutting needle #693 (Ethicon)
2	Ampules Xylocaine, HCl 1%, 2 cc. (Astra)
1	Venacath 14, 15 gauge bore, 11½″ length radiopaque tubing with needle, prepackaged, sterile (Abbott Laboratories)
	or
1	Venacath 16, 18 gauge bore, 11½″ length radiopaque tubing with needle, prepackaged, sterile (Abbott Laboratories)

Prepackaged Sterile, Disposable Table and Patient Drapes for Pelvic Exenteration
   Abdominal instrument table cover and drapes:
1   Barrier basic pack code #0480 (Johnson & Johnson) contains:
      1 outer wrapper/table cover
      1 pack wrapper/table cover
      1 Mayo stand cover
      2 drape sheets
      6 absorbent towels
      1 utility drape, nonabsorbent
1   Barrier laparotomy sheet, code #0442 (Johnson & Johnson)
1   Barrier drape sheet, code #0427 (Johnson & Johnson)
1   Steri-Drape, large, code #1070 (Minnesota Mining and Manufacturing Co.)
      Perineal instrument table cover and drapes
1   Barrier lithotomy pack (Johnson & Johnson) contains:
      1 outer wrapper/table cover
      1 pack wrapper/table cover
      4 absorbent towels
      2 nonabsorbent towel-size utility drapes
      2 lithotomy leggings
      1 under buttocks drape
      1 abdominal drape

Chapter Eight

SURGICAL TECHNIQUE

Exenterative surgery of the pelvis can be divided into various subroutines for descriptive purposes. The combination and order of the subroutines undergo some variation, depending on the location of various cancers, host variables and surgical team preferences. The standard subroutines in this text were described in SURTRAN, or surgical translation, which is a method for describing complex surgical operations as simply and accurately as possible (Cook). Each technical step of the subroutine is written in a brief and positive sentence which is punched on a Hollerith card. Printouts from the cards were made and edited, and replacement cards were made. The order of the sentences is determined to conform to the actual steps in the surgical operation, and in the editing process the statements on each card were checked against technical movements of the operating surgeon in an actual situation to avoid biases arising from the perception and memory of the surgeon. Then a final printout of the edited cards properly sequenced can be made.

SURTRAN can best be used in communication between experienced surgeons, since it presumes the commonality of basic knowledge in anatomy and methods of dissection. This commonality of knowledge reduces dependency on illustrations. When SURTRAN is used, illustrations can be restricted to points in technique that cannot be satisfactorily covered by SURTRAN or that require further emphasis. Because SURTRAN is still an experimental method for communicating surgical methods, it has been edited back into standard descriptive style in the final writing of this chapter. The detailed description of those subroutines in use by the authors is recorded. Several subroutines are not discussed because of the rarity of indications for them or because they are considered to be in common usage among surgeons and do not require detailed description. Some related subroutines are grouped together in the paragraphing of the text or are too minor to merit separate identification.

SUBROUTINES FOR EXENTERATIVE SURGERY OF THE PELVIS

1. Positioning of patient
   a. Supine, for subsequent dorsal lithotomy
   b. Supine, lower extremities abducted
   c. Supine, partial rotation for hemipelvectomy
2. Preparation
   a. Surgical setting
   b. Skin
   c. Intestines
   d. Bladder
3. Draping
4. Incisions
   a. Decisions
   b. Midline
   c. Transverse
   d. Colostomy
   e. Ileal segment
   f. Perineal
   g. Hemipelvectomy
5. Exploration
6. Exposure
7. Lateral pelvic dissection
   a. Total exenteration
   b. Anterior exenteration
   c. Posterior exenteration
8. Presacral dissection
9. Retropubic dissection
10. Vesicovaginal dissection
11. Rectovaginal dissection
12. Retroprostatic dissection
13. Perineal dissection
   a. Total exenteration
   b. Anterior exenteration
   c. Posterior exenteration
14. Drainage
15. Closure
   a. Abdomen
   b. Pelvis
16. Modification for en bloc inclusion of other organs
   a. Hemicorporectomy
   b. Hemipelvectomy
   c. Vulvectomy
   d. Ischiectomy
   e. Groin dissections

17. Reconstructive procedures
    a. Ileal segment
    b. Colostomy
    c. Neovagina
18. Special techniques
    a. Control of hemorrhage
    b. Packing
    c. Drainage
    d. Dressing

POSITIONING THE PATIENT

The arrangement of the operating room table and the proper position and draping of a patient are shown in Figures 8–1 and 8–2. This position (supine with lower extremities abducted) is used routinely at EFSCH for most total exenterations of the pelvis and the operations

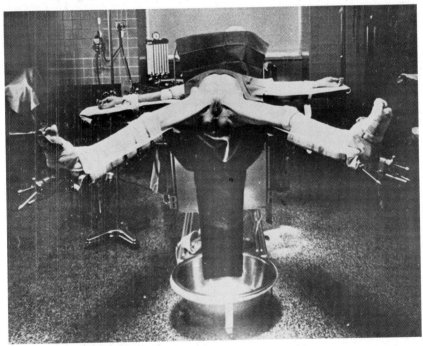

Figure 8–1 The patient is positioned on the operating table with leg traction units mounted. The screw clamps for the leg traction have been tightened to hold both lower extremities in widely abducted position during subsequent inguinal and perineal operations. (From Spratt, J. S., Jr., Donegan, W. L., and Rapp, M.: Positioning and some variations in surgical technique used for combined inguinal, perineal, and abdominal cancer surgery. Am. J. Obstet. Gynecol., 99:417, 1967.)

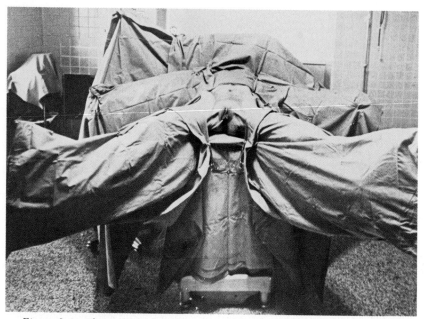

Figure 8–2 The patient is shown from a distance after preparation and sterile draping. (From Spratt, J. S., Jr., Donegan, W. L., and Rapp, M.: Positioning and some variations in surgical technique used for combined inguinal, perineal, and abdominal cancer surgery. Am. J. Obstet. Gynecol., 99:417, 1967.)

listed in Table 8–1 not requiring movement of the lower extremities during surgery. When the position shown in Figure 8–1 is used, the sacrum must be well padded to avoid pressure sores (Spratt, 1967).

Alternately, the lower extremities can be placed on the lower portion of the operating table, and the abduction attachments can be omitted. This arrangement provides flexibility of exposure needed for various subroutines of exenterative operations, such as the simultaneous performance of hemipelvectomy or the need for the dorsal lithotomy or Sims's position for exposure of the coccygeal or sacral regions when the proximity of the neoplasm requires that posterior areas be accessible to insure an adequate posterior margin around the neoplasm.

PREPARATION OF THE OPERATIVE SITE

After the induction of endotracheal anesthesia, the skin is shaved and prepared with a Septisol scrub, and Betadine solution is applied from the nipples to the knees, including the inner thighs and the perineum.

Table 8–1   Surgical Table Positions for Different Exenterative
Surgical Procedures of the Pelvis

POSITION	SURGICAL PROCEDURE
Supine with lower extremities abducted on orthopedic extensions	Bilateral groin dissection vulvectomy
	Radical penectomy and bilateral groin dissection
	Anterior pelvic exenteration
	Total pelvic exenteration
	Radical abdominoperineal cystectomy (an anterior pelvic exenteration)
	Wertheim hysterectomy
	Contraindications to position, posterior pelvic exenteration, abdominoperineal resection, conjoined hemipelvectomy, need for coccygeal or sacral resection.
Supine with shift to dorsal lithotomy or Sims's position for perineal dissection	Abdominoperineal dissection of the rectum; posterior pelvic exenteration, preferred for any exenteration requiring coccygeal or sacral exposure
Supine with abdominal, perineal, gluteal and extremity preparation; with sterile draping under patient from lumbar spine caudally, and with distal part of extremity to be moved, draped from the midthigh to include the feet; the extremity, hip and pelvis can then be manipulated as necessary for the gluteal incision and flap elevation and osseous transection near the sacroiliac joint	Pelvic exenteration and hemipelvectomy

A Foley urinary catheter is inserted and left in place. It is attached to a sterile drainage system in order to keep the bladder empty during the pelvic dissection. A Pezzer catheter is next placed in the rectal ampulla and is sutured to the anal skin. The Pezzer catheter is attached to closed drainage to keep the rectal ampulla empty.

The positioning of the table, patient and drapes is shown in Figures 8–1 and 8–2. During the abdominal exploration, the perineum is covered with two sterile towels.

INCISIONS

The type and location of the incision is determined in part by the condition of the anterior abdominal wall. Scars from previous surgical operations and the location of entry and exit ports from previous external radiation influence the location of incisions. After aseptic preparation of the abdominal skin and before the sterile drapes are applied, the gowned and gloved surgeon marks the locations of all abdominal incisions and all potential stomata. It is particularly important to cut a superficial cross mark in the skin at the center point of the planned sites of colostomies and ileostomies. This center point, generally located halfway between the umbilicus and the anterior superior iliac spine, must be situated so that it will allow a ring of normal skin around the stoma large enough to accommodate the application of an ileostomy bag. These bags will not adhere to irregular surfaces, old scars or bony prominences. Also, previously irradiated skin may ulcerate and necrose in the presence of the stoma or after the application of the bag.

A lower midline abdominal incision is the most desirable. Such incisions should avoid irradiated abdominal wall when possible. If much of the central pelvic radiation has been given by high energy external pelvic techniques using abutting or overlapping suprapubic ports, the incision necessarily must be made through irradiated tissues. In such instances the patient must accept the increased risk of poor wound healing. There is little, if any, place for the transverse lower abdominal incision in the performance of exenterative operations in the pelvis. To obtain adequate deep pelvic exposure, the lower midline abdominal incision should extend from 2 cm. above the umbilicus to the pubic symphysis. Should the upper end of the incision extend further into the epigastrium, subsequent packing of the intestines out of the pelvis will be more difficult because the lax abdominal wall will not retain the packs in place. Similarily, mobilization of the pelvic viscera will be more difficult and the pelvic structures less exposed if the lower end of the incision does not expose the edge of the pubic symphysis.

After the incision has been made, exploration of the abdominal and pelvic cavity is carried out.

EXPLORATION

An extremely careful exploration of the opened abdomen is necessary before proceeding with exenterative surgery in the pelvis. The sites requiring careful scouting are the liver and the periaortic and renal lymph node–bearing areas. These must be examined by palpation from the diaphragmatic hiatus to the aortic bifurcation. Unusually firm lymph nodes are the culprits sought. Enlargement is also important, but a lymph node containing metastatic cancer becomes firm before enlarging. Suspicious lymph nodes outside the field of pelvic dissection should be excised and submitted to frozen section examination to exclude the presence of extrapelvic cancer.

The liver must be examined with equal care; any area thought to be metastatic should be checked by biopsy before concluding that the patient is incurable by resective surgery. Since the liver is generally examined through a lower abdominal incision, this biopsy may not be as simple as it would be through an upper abdominal incision. The poor exposure can be overcome by taking a Silverman needle biopsy through the upper abdominal wall. The surgeon's hand in the peritoneal cavity can direct the needle into the area for biopsy. The anesthetist can create a temporary respiratory arrest before the needle enters the liver for the biopsy lasting until the needle is removed. With careful prepositioning with a pretested needle, the respiratory arrest will be very transient.

The remainder of the exploration is a systematic palpatory examination of the remaining viscera for metastatic deposits and other indications of pathology. Other pathological conditions, such as gallstones and enlarged kidneys, should be carefully noted and *recorded in the operative note*. Although certain conditions may not deter the surgeon, they may be sources of postoperative complications, such as acute cholecystitis secondary to cholelithiasis.

Particular attention must be paid to the peritoneum and omentum. Both may be foci of small implantation metastases or of a more diffuse thickening produced by retroperitoneal spread. Suspicious foci should be subjected to biopsy for frozen section examination.

To examine the pelvis adequately, the small intestines and omentum must be delivered from the pelvic cavity. The intestines are held out of the cavity temporarily by an assistant while the pelvis is explored by the surgeon and the extent of the neoplasm is determined. The only categorical contraindication to resection at this point is extension of the cancer out of the true pelvis. Should the mass seem to extend to the lateral pelvic wall, it is sometimes wise to explore the obturator fossa and the region lateral to the external iliac vessels to determine if extension into the psoas muscle has occurred before making the final decision regarding operability.

Another exploratory maneuver which is often helpful in defining the lateral extent of the tumor is the mobilization of the urinary bladder from the symphysis pubis and the rectum from the anterior surface of the sacrum. This permits better assessment of the mobility and lateral extent of the tumor and may avoid the surgical mistake of having undertaken the exenterative procedure only to find out the lesion is inoperable after transection of ureters and colon. With the information obtained from this exploration, the surgeon is in a position to decide upon the type of exenterative operation indicated. If the surgeon elects to perform a total exenteration, the next subroutine is the performance of an end sigmoid colostomy with closure of the proximal end of the distal sigmoid colon.

Complete exposure of the pelvic organs is essential to the performance of any type of exenteration. Obtaining this exposure is prerequisite to beginning the pelvic dissection. When a total exenteration is to be performed, the sigmoid colostomy is constructed before the pelvic dissection is begun (see section on Colostomy later in this chapter). Upon completion of the colostomy, the surgeon is ready to begin the pelvic dissection. The closed distal sigmoid is replaced into the pelvis temporarily, and the small intestines are retracted into the upper abdomen. Three lap gauzes (16″ square) are used to maintain the upper abdominal position of the small intestines and cecum. The cecum is partially mobilized and is held cephalad with the folded edge of a laparotomy gauze under another Deaver retractor.

Next, the edges of the wound are covered with gauze and a Balfour retractor is inserted. After this retractor has been widely spread to retract the abdominal wall adequately, a medium or long center piece is attached, depending on the dorsoventral depth of the abdomen, and this is retracted cephalad against a laparotomy gauze. The Deaver retractors are removed as this is done. If the laparotomy gauzes have been properly placed, no further retraction is necessary to maintain the small intestines in the upper abdomen. Finally, a 5- to 10-degree Trendelenburg position may be helpful and may be requested before the intestinal packing is done.

A note of caution concerning packing of the intestines into the upper abdomen needs to be made. If too much packing or too much force is applied, one may encounter physiological changes due to abnormally elevated diaphragms, occlusion of the hepatic veins or inferior venae cavae, impaired blood flow to intestines and compression of the aorta and/or vena cava by the central blade of the self-retaining retractor. Careful positioning of packs and retractors is more important than great force in seeking necessary exposure. These adverse effects should be suspected in any patient who develops a sustained or unexplained hypotension after the packs are in place. Should hypotension develop, the packs should be removed promptly. If they were the cause of the hypotension, the blood pressure should rise immediately. The repacking should be performed more carefully, slowly and less forcefully. Should the small intestines escape from the upper abdomen during the operation, the situation is best handled by removing all gauze and repacking, since nonsystematic improvisation of intestinal packing is rarely successful in maintaining adequate exposure.

LATERAL PELVIC DISSECTION

The approach to the lateral pelvic dissection is determined in part by the type of exenteration to be performed. For example, a presacral dissection is unnecessary with an anterior exenteration. Since various combinations of dissections are determined by the peculiarities of individual neoplasms, the different dissections will be described as separate subroutines.

For total or posterior exenterations, the presacral dissection is the starting point. The distal sigmoid colon is elevated, and the presacral space is entered at the base of the mesosigmoid. Under direct vision, divide the attachments between the mesosigmoid, rectum and the sacrum. Continue blunt and sharp dissection to the tip of the coccyx. Stay anterior to the presacral veins. These may be seen by retracting the rectum and sigmoid ventrally to expose the presacral space for the sharp transection of the avascular rectal mesentery.

In a total exenteration the bladder is usually detached from its anterior peritoneal and retropubic attachments before the lateral dissection is undertaken. The retropubic dissection is performed by applying gentle cephalad and dorsal traction to the dome of the bladder. This permits the surgeon to identify the avascular prevesical space. In this space, the bladder is easily reflected from the pubis by gentle, blunt dissection. Care should be taken to avoid injuring the periurethral vascular plexus near the urogenital diaphragm. Should injury to the plexus occur, the bleeding is best controlled temporarily by packing. The entire plexus will be resected subsequently.

When only an anterior exenteration is being performed, detachment of the bladder is delayed until the vesicorectal or rectovaginal space has been dissected. The delay facilitates exposure by having the bladder held forward with its own natural attachments during the dissection.

Stepwise dissection involves the incision of the peritoneum and pelvic fascia along and down to the fibers of the psoas muscle just medial to the genitofemoral nerve. The testicular or ovarian vessels and the round ligament are identified, clamped, transected and ligated as they are encountered along the pelvic brim.

The ureters are transected 1 inch distal to the crossing of the external iliac artery. The ureters are always ligated distally. The proximal ends are ligated whenever the urine is thought to be or to have been recently infected. The pelvic fascia is reflected from the psoas muscle to the lateral side of the external iliac artery.

The fascia forming the anterior vascular sheath is then reflected medially from ventral surface of the external iliac artery and veins. With a sponge stick on the external iliac vein to roll it laterally, the pelvic fascia is reflected from the dorsal surface of the vessels to the obturator internus muscle. The pelvic fascia covering the obturator internus (the obturator fascia) is continuous with the external iliac vascular sheath.

The pelvic fascia is reflected from this muscle caudally to the arcus tendineus, marking the origin of the levator ani muscle. The obturator nerve that comes from beneath the upper psoas through the parietal layer of the pelvic fascia can be seen through and adjacent to this fascia.

To preserve the obturator nerve, the pelvic fascia is incised over the nerve, and the nerve is reflected laterally by dissecting it from its fascial attachments. Hold the nerve laterally with a vein retractor until all pelvic fascia has been reflected away from the obturator internus down to the arcus tendineus.

Next, identify the obturator vein and artery passing through the obturator foramen. Cross clamp these vessels with hemoclips, and transect between clips. If hemoclips are not available, silk ligatures can be individually passed about the vessels with a right angle clamp and tied. The thin walls of the obturator artery and vein will not tolerate the trauma and traction of a hemostat. If these vessels are torn at the obturator foramen, they may retract into the thigh, making hemostasis difficult. The obturator foramen must be oversewn with 0 chromic catgut ligatures and swaged on a general closure needle should this vascular retraction occur with continued hemorrhage.

Separately, pass a right angle clamp carefully deep or lateral to the internal iliac artery to permit passage of a 2–0 silk ligature around the vessel. Care must be taken to avoid the superior gluteal artery that originates on the deep or lateral surface of the internal iliac artery near the origin of the latter. Repeat the ligation distally at least 1 cm. Pass a 2–0 silk suture through the artery and suture ligate proximally. Transect the internal iliac artery between the proximal suture ligature and the distal tie.

When bladder attachments are to be transected, the peritoneal incision lateral to the external iliac vessels and medial to the genitofemoral nerve is extended toward the internal abdominal ring and on to the lower edge of the midline abdominal incision. This lower end of the abdominal incision must always divide the rectus fascia to the pubic symphysis. Staying adjacent the pubic periosteum, the areolar tissue in the prevesical space is dissected away from the pelvic side of the pubis.

At this point, the lymphatic cord passing from the thigh can be identified. This cord is composed of fatty areolar tissue containing the major valvular lymphatics connecting the iliac and femoral lymphatics. The cord passes through the inguinopectineal triangle medial to the external iliac vein. The cord should be ligated adjacent the inguinopectineal triangle to prevent possible lymph fistulas and lymphoceles from the large volume of lymph that will flow from the lower extremity into the pelvic wound (Spratt, 1965).

After the internal iliac artery is transected, the internal iliac vein is usually visible. Previously, the pelvic fascia has been dissected away from the musculoskeletal pelvis on the two opposite sides of the internal iliac vein during the exposure of the presacral space and the obturator internus muscle. How the balance of the lateral pelvic dissection is completed now depends on the condition of the perivenous tissues. In the presence of fibrosis residual from previous radiation or pelvic infection, or when a large primary cancer or enlarged iliac lymph nodes preclude satisfactory exposure of the vein, individual identification of the venous branches may prove tedious, difficult and dangerous. Under these circumstances the risk of entering these veins is great, resulting in rapid and massive hemorrhage.

Before proceeding, the branches of the sciatic nerve or lumbosacral plexus must be seen. The lumbosacral trunk, composed of the fourth and fith lumbar nerve roots, is situated dorsal and lateral to the obturator nerve lying adjacent the caudal fibers of the obturator internus. Once this trunk has been identified, the other sacral roots should be avoided by continuing the dissection medially and downward.

When the extent of fibrosis precludes the individual dissection of the internal iliac vascular tree, the tissue medial to the sacral plexus can still be developed by digital dissection into three bundles con-

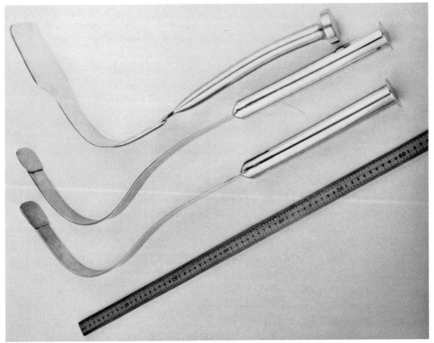

Figure 8-3 Bricker retractors.

taining the superior gluteal vessels, the inferior gluteal vessels, and the internal pudendal vessels. These bundles are individually clamped with 12″ Viet-Harrington clamps placed with the convex curve of the clamp parallel to the inward curve of the musculoskeletal pelvis, avoiding the lumbosacral nerve plexus. Space usually limits the surgeon to the placement of a single clamp on each bundle. Occasionally, an unusually roomy pelvis may permit the placement of two clamps on each bundle, but this is not a necessity, since back bleeding from the specimen can be controlled by pressure from a deep pelvic retractor especially designed for this purpose by Bricker (Fig. 8–3). The retractor simultaneously holds the specimen, medially giving better lateral pelvic exposure, and controls back bleeding from the specimen by direct pressure.

With the specimen retracted medially, the clamped bundles are individually oversown with a running swaged-on 0 chromic catgut suture on a general closure needle before the clamps are removed. Each suture is pulled taut after the clamp is removed, and the ends are then tied. This suturing is performed with the 12″ long needle holders.

A variation in the placement of these sutures which is quite effective in the prevention of bleeding entails the insertion of the suture through the midportion of the bundle initially; the needle is next passed through the distal edge of the bundle which should be just proximal to the point of the Viet-Harrington clamps. Finally, it is passed through the proximal portion. The needle is then cut from the suture, and a single loop is placed in the suture in readiness to draw the loop taut on the vascular bundle as the clamp is removed. The square knot is then completed.

In recent years, the availabililty of Weck hemoclips has simplified the completion of the lateral pelvic dissection. When the lateral pelvic fascia can be dissected from the veins easily, the veins may be secured with a double layer of hemoclips followed by transection of the vessels between the clips. Alternately, two Viet-Harrington clamps can be placed on the previously described bundles. The clamp adjacent to the pelvic wall can then be removed, and large Weck clips are progressively placed on this crushed tissue. The tissue is then divided adjacent to the medial clamp.

After the vascular bundles have been transected, the dissection is carried downward and medially across the pelvic side of the levator ani muscle. The extent of the dissection along the pelvic surface of the levator ani muscle is determined by the lateral extent of the neoplasm.

ANTERIOR PELVIC EXENTERATION

When the decision is made to perform an anterior pelvic exenteration, the operative procedure varies in the following ways. In women the anterior exenteration may be done in three different planes, depending on the nature of the neoplasm, i.e., rectovaginal, transvaginal and vesicovaginal. In men only the rectoprostatic plane exists for the performance of anterior pelvic exenteration. Experience with this dissection is best acquired by preceptorial training with a surgeon experienced in pelvic surgery. Understanding the levels of dissection requires careful study of the fascial anatomy described in the anatomy chapter (see Chap. Two).

When the anterior vaginal wall is to be removed with the specimen, the posterior vaginal fornix must be entered, and the lateral vaginal walls must be transected down to the vaginal outlet. The vagina is composed of erectile tissue that bleeds freely. Consequently, this step should be delayed until the specimen has been mobilized to the point that it is nearly ready for removal. The reason for this is that a running 0 chromic catgut suture (usually locked) must be placed along the cut edge of the vagina to secure hemostasis. The best exposure for this is obtained when the specimen is removed. The hemostatic suture may then be placed through either the abdominal or the perineal wound, depending on the surgeon's preference. Rarely is the remaining vagina large enough to permit anterior approximation of the cut edges with reconstruction of a functional vagina.

Unless the extent of the cancer, usually cancer of the bladder, merits removal of the anterior vaginal wall, it is usually preferable to enter the vesicovaginal space and dissect the anterior vaginal wall away from the bladder and urethra down to the vaginal outlet.

More frequently, anterior exenteration is indicated in males with large bladder cancers. This necessitates entry into the prostaticorectal space and dissection of the rectum away from the rectovesical septum, formerly called Denonvilliers' fascia. This requires good exposure and careful dissection to avoid rectal perforation. The long scissor points should always be turned anteriorly, and the fascial attachments that must be transected should be cut against the prostatic fascia. When the specimen has been removed from the pelvis, the rectal wall must always be inspected very carefully. This requires placement of the index finger through the anus to stretch the anterior rectal wall for direct visual inspection. Perforations must be repaired by a double layer of inverting sutures. A proximal loop sigmoid colostomy is required when this complication occurs. The colostomy is not closed until the perineal wound is well healed.

When the anterior exenteration is being performed for bladder cancer in the female, the urethra is removed en bloc with the bladder. In the male, the penile urethra is exposed through a ventral penile incision from the meatus to the perineum. As a precaution against implantation metastases, the bladder and urethra are irrigated with 10 per cent formalin after exploration of the abdomen and pelvis has established that all gross cancer is restricted to the region that will permit complete removal by anterior exenteration (Long).

COLOSTOMY

The colostomy most frequently used for total exenterative surgery is an end colostomy structured from the midsigmoid colon. It is usually performed after a positive decision, based on the exploratory findings, has been made to perform the exenteration. Elevate sigmoid colon from the left lower quadrant and examine the mesosigmoid for presence of enlarged lymph nodes or blood vessels that should be considered during the mesenteric division. Identify the point of colonic transection at a point on normal sigmoid that will allow enough mobility of proximal colon for the transected end to traverse the abdominal wall and reach the abdominal skin without traction. Identify both ureters and avoid traction or injury of them. Incise the peritoneum of the sigmoid mesocolon and the vascular branches of it from promontory of the sacrum to contemplated point of sigmoid transection. Only for sigmoid, rectal or anal cancer is it desirable to transect the inferior mesenteric artery near its origin from the aorta. The inferior mesenteric vein is ligated and transected at the same level as the artery.

Identify the cross mark on the abdominal skin placed previously, usually halfway between the umbilicus and the anterior superior iliac spine. Place a Rochester-Ochsner clamp in skin at center of the cross mark and elevate. Make a circular incision in skin approximately 1½ inch in diameter. Remove the full thickness of the circularly incised area of skin (Fig. 8–4). Take care now to insure that all layers of the abdominal wall are incised so that the final hole through all layers will be straight when the abdominal incision is closed at the completion of the operation. To do this, place a Rochester-Ochsner clamp on the fascia and a towel clip in the skin edge at the midline abdominal incision and place both the Rochester-Ochsner clamp and the towel clip on uniform tension. Cross-cut the fascia and muscles to make a full thickness hole through the abdominal wall at the same level as the circular skin incision. A pulse is usually palpable in the inferior epigastric artery; this permits the surgeon to avoid it. Should these vessels be cut accidently, the surgeon must open the peritoneum sufficiently to secure and ligate the bleeding vessel. Hemostasis should be complete throughout this incision before the colon is brought through it.

The tip of a large Payr clamp is next passed through this circular incision in the abdominal wall (from the skin side). This clamp is then used to cross clamp the sigmoid colon just proximal to the previously selected point for colonic transection. The proximal end of the tran-

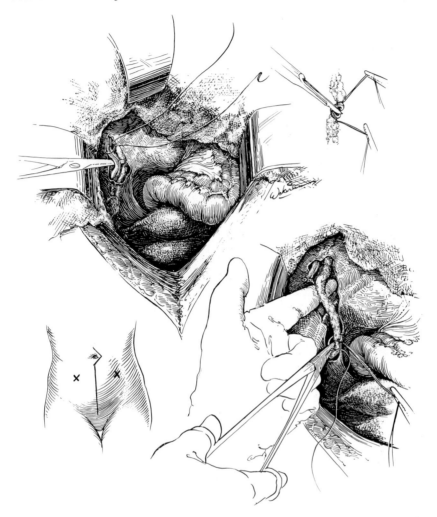

Figure 8–4 The planned location of stomata must be indelibly marked on the patient's skin before anatomical landmarks are covered by surgical drapes. The stomata are most often centered half way between the umbilicus and the anterior superior iliac spine. The occasional presence of old surgical scars or radiation ports requires selection of other sites. The site selected should have a band of normal skin surface. The incision of choice is suprapubic midline.

After abdominal and pelvic exploration has been performed as described in the text, and the decision has been made that an ileal segment will be constructed, the ureters are mobilized, ligated and transected. The most desirable point for transection is 2 cm. caudal to the point at which the ureters cross the iliac vessels.

sected sigmoid colon held by this Payr clamp will then be delivered through the abdominal wall after transection. The distal colon is cross clamped with a second small Payr clamp placed parallel with and adjacent to the more proximal clamp. The colon is transected between these two Payr clamps. A 2–0 chromic running Connell suture is then placed in the distal colon over the distal Payr clamp. As the clamp is removed, the Connell suture is tied to occlude and invert the distal colon. This occluded end is then placed into the pelvis for subsequent removal with the specimen through the perineal incision.

Before the proximal colon end is brought through the abdominal wall, sutures are placed to obliterate the peritoneal space lateral to the sigmoid mesocolon. This left peritoneal gutter must be closed to avoid later internal hernias. An 0 chromic catgut suture swaged on a general closure needle is held in a long needle holder (8–10''). A continuous suture is placed around the left lateral peritoneal gutter, running from the left peritoneal edge of the circular abdominal incision down the lateral abdominal wall to the cut edge of the sigmoid mesentery and up along the peritoneal edge of the transected mesocolon. The last pass of the needle is through the peritoneum of the sigmoid mesentery at a distance from the cut edge of the colon equivalent to the thickness of the abdominal wall. The Payr clamp and the proximal end of the transected colon are then withdrawn through the circular incision.

The handle of the Payr clamp is then fixed with a towel clip placed across the handle and into the drapes so as to avoid rotation or traction upon the colon. Cover the colon end with a dry laparotomy gauze and secure to avoid exposure during subsequent phases of the operation.

Finally, tie the 0 chromic catgut suture placed around the lateral peritoneal gutter just tight enough to close the space between the proximal cut end of the sigmoid mesocolon and the peritoneum of the left lateral gutter. The open end of the colostomy will be sutured to the skin after the abdominal incision is closed by the same technique described for suturing the urinary ileal conduit to the skin (Fig. 8–14).

ILEAL BLADDER

The ileal bladder may be constructed in varying sequences with the other subroutines. If the distal ureters are partially or totally obstructed from the pelvic cancer, the proximal urinary tract may be infected, the renal function is below its maximum functional capacity and the patient may have obstructive azotemia. In this situation the ileal segment is constructed before the pelvic exenteration is performed. When the infection or azotemia is severe, the total operation is often staged and only the ileal segment or ileal segment and colostomy are performed, and the patient is permitted to recuperate. The time interval between stages should be no shorter than two weeks to permit physiological recuperation. During this period, pelvic and urinary tract infections are treated actively, and urinary output is maintained at a volume adequate to correct the azotemia. The time interval between stages should rarely be allowed to exceed six weeks because pelvic adhesions can become quite dense and vascular within this period, making pelvic dissection difficult and in some cases impossible.

In most total exenterations the ileal segment is not constructed until the perineal dissection is completed, the specimen is removed and the perineal defect is closed or is being closed by an assistant. Gauze packs are used to fill the pelvis during construction of the ileal conduit. They absorb any lymph or blood, vascular oozing and the urine egressing from the ureters. Also, the packs help hold the ileum and cecum in the surgical field for easier access.

When the ileal bladder is to be constructed, the laparotomy packs used to keep the intestine in the upper abdomen during the pelvic dissection are removed. The cecum and terminal ileum are then deliv-

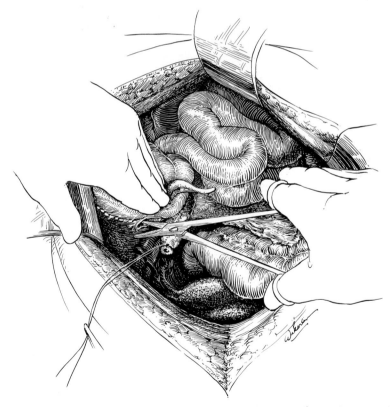

Figure 8–5 The cecum is next mobilized by transecting the peritoneum at its base and along its lateral gutter. After the ileal segment has been constructed, this mobilized cecum will be brought medial to the mesentery of the ileal segment.

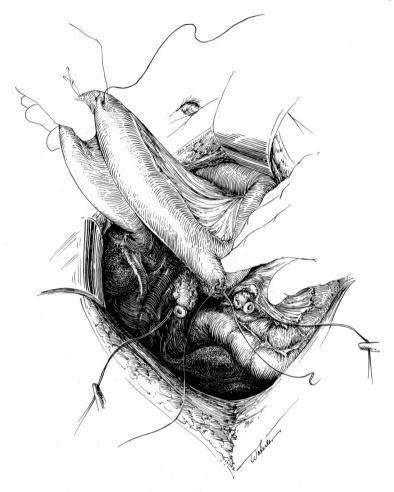

Figure 8–6   The length of the ileal segment is determined by the distance needed to traverse the distance between the sacral promontory and the skin of the anterior abdominal wall without traction or redundancy. The length selected should also be adequate to permit eversion of the distal end of the ileum as shown in Figure 8–14. The length can be permanently identified by placing marking sutures in the serosa.

The proximal end of the left ureter has been brought through the tunnel made at the base of the sigmoid mesocolon. When the sigmoid mesocolon has been transected in preparation for a total exenteration the left ureter simply passes to the right side just caudal to the transected edge of the sigmoid mesocolon.

ered into the wound. Partial mobilization of the right colon improves access to the ileum (Fig. 8–5). The segment of ileum to be used as the ileal urinary conduit is identified (Fig. 8–8). This is accomplished by transillumination of the vasculature in the mesentery of a 6- to 8-inch segment of terminal ileum. This mesentery should contain at least two major arteries feeding a more distal mesenteric vascular arcade. An arterial branch of the arcade should reach the ileum at a distance no greater than 1 cm. from the ends of the divided ileum. Should the terminal ileum be altered by severe adhesions or scarring secondary to radiation, the involved segment must generally be excised. The intestine to be used in the ileal conduit is then isolated from the normal small intestine just proximal to the resected segment of abnormal bowel. By doing so, only one enteroenterostomy is necessary, and this anastomosis is near the cecum.

The artist's drawings of the ileal segment construction (Figs. 8–4 to 8–15) depict the operation in the presence of an intact sigmoid mesocolon. When the sigmoid mesocolon is not transected, the surgeon, after inspection of the vasculature of the sigmoid mesocolon,

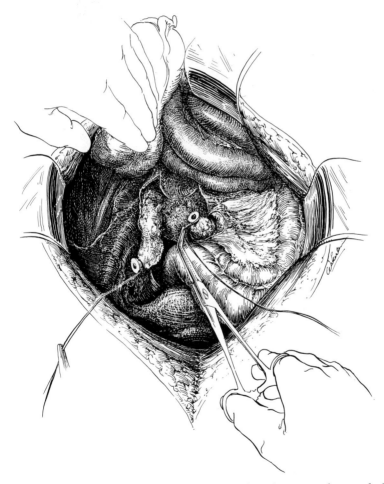

Figure 8–7 The right angle clamp is shown pulling the proximal cut end of the left ureter through a tunnel that has been dissected through the mesentery at the base of the sigmoid mesocolon at a point caudal and dorsal to the inferior mesenteric artery and vein.

Text continued on page 118.

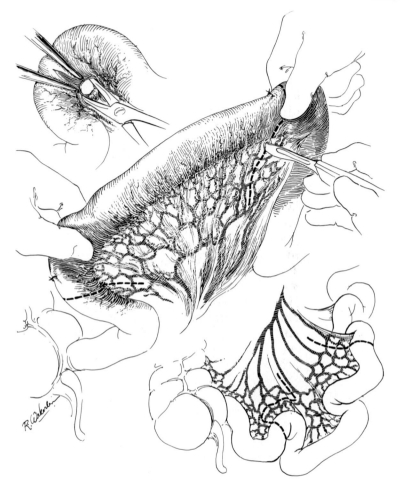

Fig. 8-8

Figures 8-8 and 8-9   After the gross length of the intestine has been marked, the mesentery must be held up for transillumination to identify the location of the mesenteric blood vessels. The peritoneum on either side of the mesentery is incised and the intervening fat is spread with a scissors or a hemostat. The object is to ensure accurate hemostasis of blood vessels that must be transected and ligated and to ensure that an intact vascular arcade remains at the base of the ileal segment's mesentery. An end vessel from the arcade should go within 1 cm. of each end of the segment.

After this dissection has been done the points at which the intestine must be transected are obvious. The intestine is transected between Dennis clamps, as shown. The proximal end is closed with a 3-0 chromic running Connell suture over the Dennis clamp. When the clamp has been removed the Connell suture is reversed. A final row of interrupted silk mattress sutures is then placed.

In an extremely obese individual, the mesentery at the distal end of the segment has to be incised as shown in the lower right illustration in Figure 8-8.

Finally the proximal end of the segment is folded with its mesentery to the base of the mesentery. To close the potential space for an internal hernia, fine silk sutures (interrupted) are placed between the peritoneum on either side of the space (Fig. 8-9).

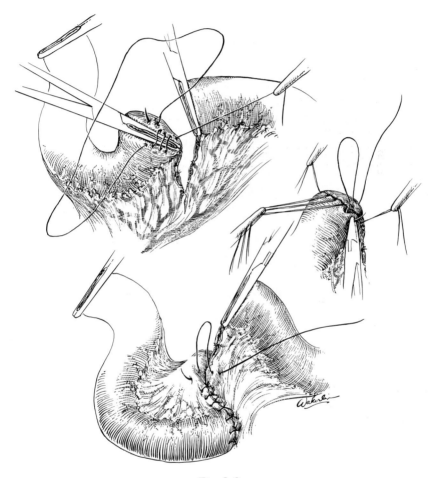

Fig. 8–9

See opposite page for legend.

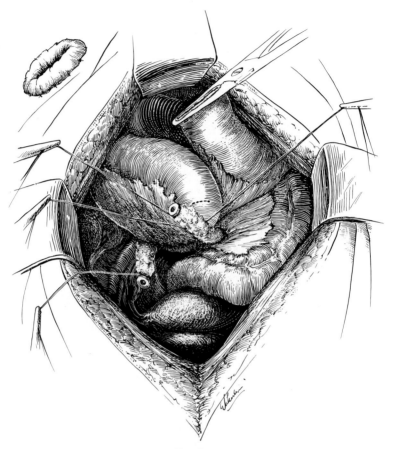

Fig. 8-10

Figures 8–10, 8–11 and 8–12   The two ureters are being sutured to the base of the ileal mesentery and proximal end of the ileum up to the point selected for ureteroileal anastomosis. Each suture is 5–0 silk between the adventitia of the ureter and the peritoneum of the mesentery or ileum. The last two silk sutures at the point of anastomosis are left long for traction and stability. Just before the anastomosis is started, the distal end of each ureter is transected with fine scissors to remove that ureter crushed by the tie or other instrument handling. The proximal end of the ureter remaining is never held in a potentially crushing instrument after this transection.

The seromuscular layer of the ileum is then incised at the point of anastomosis with a no. 11 blade. The pointed blade is used to tease the ileal mucosa into the incision. This mucosa must be kept from retracting until transfixed by the first suture.

The ureter is then anastomosed to the ileum with 5–0 chromic catgut suture swaged on to fine vascular needles. Each suture passes through all layers of ureter and all layers of ileum. Small ureters may be held open with vascular pickups placed within the lumen, avoiding any crush. No more than four or five sutures are needed for small ureters. Finally the adventitia of the ureter is approximated to the serosa of the ileum with several 5–0 silk sutures.

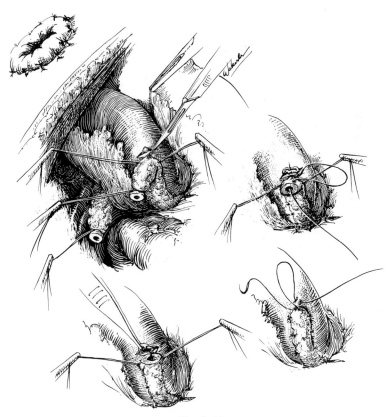

Fig. 8–11

See opposite page for legend.

selects an avascular area caudal and dorsal to the inferior mesenteric artery and vein. The peritoneum of both sides of the mesocolon is sharply incised at this point. The fat of the mesocolon is then gently spread to establish a connecting tunnel. The surgeon then passes a right angle clamp through this avascular tunnel from right to left. Either the suture on the end of the ureter or the adventitia near the tip of the ureter is grasped with the top of the right angle clamp, and the left ureter is brought through the avascular tunnel. To avoid retraction of the ureters back through the tunnel, a 5-0 black silk suture is passed through the adventitia of the ureter and the peritoneum of the mesocolon and is tied. Before fixing the ureter with this suture, as much

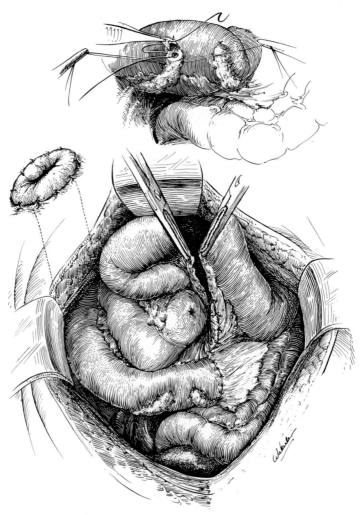

Fig. 8-12

See page 116 for legend.

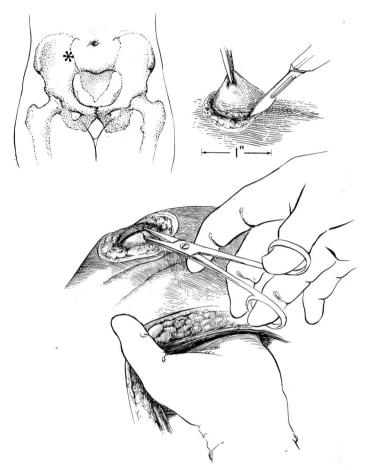

Figure 8–13 The incisions for both the ileostomy and colostomy must be circular. For factors that must be considered in selecting stomal location, see pp. 99–100. At the center point of the stomal site the skin is grasped with a clamp and is retracted upward. While the skin is held, the circular incision is marked off lightly with the scalpel. When circularity is adequate, the incision is extended full thickness through the skin. The diameter of the removed circle of skin should be 1″.

Then the deep abdominal fascia is transected as shown. The muscle is spread and the transverse fascia and peritoneum are then transected. Two fingers should traverse the incision with ease and without contacting restrictive fascial bands (Fig. 8–12).

ureter as can be brought through the tunnel without traction or kinking should be accessible for the subsequent left ureteroileal anastomosis.

After a segment of the small intestine has been chosen for the ileal conduit the stomal, or distal, end of the segment is isolated by transecting the ileum and the subjacent mesentery between small intestinal clamps so that an adequate length of mesentery exists to permit the end of the segment to pass through the abdominal wall

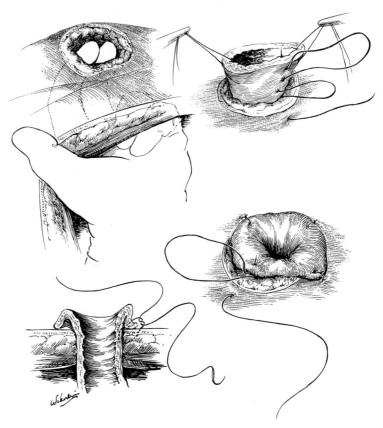

Figure 8–14   The ends of both the ileum and the colon are approximated to the skin with the same suture. Either interrupted fine silk or fine catgut sutures are placed by traversing skin and the seromuscular layer of the intestine about 1 cm. proximal to end and full thickness at the cut end of the intestine.

without tension (Figs. 8–6 and 8–8). The placement of the stomal end must avoid compromise of the mesenteric intestinal vasculature by traction. The proximal end of the segment is next transected between clamps, and the mesentery is divided for a short distance. The distance must be sufficient to permit end-to-end ileoileal anastomosis without kinking or tension. The shorter the incision in the mesentery, the greater the collateral blood supply to the isolated ileal segment.

When the patient is obese, it may be necessary to cut the mesentery parallel to the long axis of the distal segment. This permits vascularized length of ileum adequate to reach the skin without tension. The obesity also requires that the segment of ileum be longer to traverse the thicker abdominal wall (Fig. 8–8).

The proximal end of the ileal segment is then closed with running

3–0 chromic Connell sutures followed by the placement of an outer row of inverting interrupted fine silk mattress sutures (Fig. 8–9).

An end-to-end ileoileostomy is then completed with interrupted mucosal and seromuscular layers of fine silk cephalad to the segment (Fig. 8–15). The remaining rent in the mesentery can be closed with several fine silk sutures at this point or after the segment is completed (Fig. 8–9).

The proximal end of the segment is next sutured to the mesentery with several interrupted fine silk sutures to close the aperture created between the folds of the mesentery. These preceding steps can also

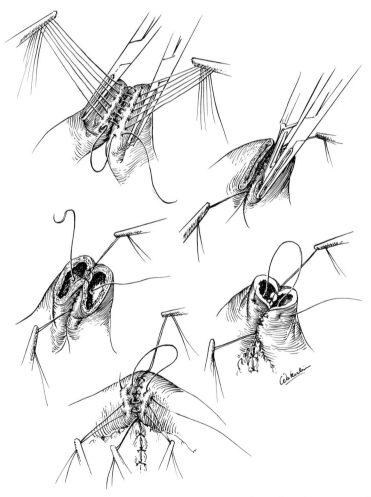

Figure 8–15 The end-to-end ileoileostomy is performed with interrupted fine silk sutures as shown. Continuous sutures are never used in end-to-end small intestinal anastomoses because of the risk of stricture. The mesentery is approximated with interrupted fine silk sutures to reduce chance of internal hernia.

be done subsequent to the ureteroileal anastomoses if the surgeon prefers. The important thing is to avoid redundant ureter that may kink when the segment is lying in its final anatomical position. It is also vital to insure that no rotation of the ureter about its long axis occurs.

Among the authors there are minor variations in the technique for performing the ureteroileal anastomoses. The steps in common are mucosa-to-mucosa sutures with 4–0 or 5–0 chromicized catgut on a small, swaged-on needle. Interrupted 4–0 or 5–0 silk sutures swaged on to a fine vascular needle are used to approximate the adventitial layer of the ureter to the seromuscular layer of the intestine. Usually no more than four to seven catgut sutures are required, depending on the size of the ureter. A similar or smaller number of silk sutures is adequate.

In doing the mucosa-to-mucosa suture, the intestinal mucosa can be illusive if certain technical steps are not followed. The seromuscular layer of the ileum should be incised with a #11 Bard-Parker blade at the point of anastomosis. The length of the seromuscular incision should be equivalent to the outside diameter of the ureter. The mucosa will pouch through this incision. The protruding mucosa should then be fixed with a fine suture before it is incised (Fig. 8–12). This permits eversion of the ileal mucosa during the placement of the inner layer of anastomotic sutures. The cut end of the ureter should never be crushed with forceps. Forceps can be inserted intraluminally into the ureter when necessary to hold open or stabilize the cut edge.

The same incision through the abdominal wall can be used to accommodate both the ileal stoma and the colostomy (Fig. 8–12). The ileal stoma is delivered through the abdominal aperture after removal of the intestinal clamp. The end of the ileal segment is manually pushed through the abdominal aperture. It must be positioned without rotation or tension. Both the ileal stoma and the sigmoid stoma are sutured to the skin, as shown in Figure 8–14, after the abdominal incision has been closed to avoid contaminating the incision and the peritoneal cavity.

The mobilized cecum and right colon are positioned medially and ventral to the ileal segment. The appendix is usually removed in a routine manner either at this time or at an earlier stage, according to the surgeon's preference.

PERINEAL DISSECTION

The perineal dissection can be performed adequately in two different positions, depending on the surgeon's preference. At Barnes

Hospital the patient is repositioned into a dorsal lithotomy position after the intra-abdominal dissection is completed. At the EFSCH the position described and illustrated in Figures 8–1 and 8–2 is utilized for anterior and total exenteration. The dorsal lithotomy position gives better exposure for coccygeal and presacral dissection when required. When extreme posterior exposure is not required, the EFSCH position avoids any necessity of repositioning the patient twice during surgery and can permit both an abdominal and a perineal surgical team to work simultaneously after a single cutaneous preparation and draping.

When a total exenteration is being performed, the perineal incision extends from the base of the clitoris to behind the anus, running just lateral to the labia minora. For cancers extending low into the vagina or into the vulva or perineum, an even wider area of vulva or perineal skin should be removed, including the entire labia majora. In the male, the incision extends from the base of the scrotum. In the female, the urethra is removed en bloc with this dissection. In the male, the proximal end of the penile urethra is exposed. The male urethra is ligated and divided at this point. When operating for bladder cancer in the male, the entire urethra is dissected from the penis through a ventral penile incision. The urethra is brought through a subscrotal tunnel to maintain the contiguity of the en bloc dissection. The ventral penile incision is closed with interrupted 3–0 plain catgut. When exenteration is being performed for bladder cancer the bladder is irrigated with 10 per cent formalin via a Foley catheter as a precaution against spillage and implantation metastasis. This irrigation is carried out as soon as the decision is made to proceed with a pelvic exenteration as determined by the abdominal and pelvic exploration. Residual formalin is left in the bladder during the pelvic and perineal dissection.

The ischium is next identified by palpation, and the perineal fascia overlying the ischiorectal fat is incised medial to it. The fascia can then be reflected in an avascular plane from the medial side of the ischium. At the cephalad apex of the ischiorectal fossa is the origin of the levator ani. When the identification of the origin is complete on both sides, the surgeon is ready to detach the levator muscle from the pubic symphysis. To detach from the symphysis, the incison is made with heavy Mayo scissors by stripping the periosteum to which the muscle is attached away from the pelvic side of the pelvis. The levator ani can then be grasped between the index and long fingers and can be transected on either side of the pelvis about a finger's breadth from its origin on the arcus tendineus. When this is complete, the surgical specimen is removed through the perineum. Hemostasis is secured after the specimen is removed. Most difficulties from bleeding will originate from the cut edge of the levator ani muscle. There are generally two principal bleeding points — the transverse perineal artery and the inferior rectal artery, both arising from the internal pudendal artery in the pudendal canal. The dissection should avoid entering the pudendal canal where troublesome bleeding may be encountered.

After removal of the surgical specimen, careful examination of the raw pelvis for bleeding points is mandatory. The arteries are rarely a source of difficulty. The larger ones have been ligated and the smaller ones contract. However, the contraction hemostasis may only be transient. On the other hand, if the veins are torn or punctured, they tend to bleed persistently, particularly in the following places: (1) presacral veins, (2) the obturator vein which can contract into the obturator foramen, (3) between the sacral nerve roots from retracted branches of the internal iliac vein, (4) along the pudendal canal and (5) behind the symphysis pubis. Usually such bleeding points can be controlled with ligatures or hemoclips. Occasionally, when veins have retracted between the sacral nerve roots, it is necessary to suture through a portion of these nerves to oversew the bleeding points and control bleeding. Bleeding from the cut edge of the levator ani can be controlled when necessary with a running, locked 0 chromic catgut suture placed in the length of the cut edge.

One patient, early in the series, died of hemorrhage because of failure to control bleeding from an obturator vein which retracted into the obturator canal. In such instances, the surgeon must secure adequate hemostasis by oversewing the foramen with an occlusive suture placed into the muscle on either side of the foramen.

In an occasional patient persistent hemorrhage may develop from the deep pelvic vessels that can be controlled only by proper gauze packing. Early recognition of the need for packing prevents further serious blood loss.

When gauze packs are left in the pelvis they become saturated with proteinaceous drainage and blood. When secondarily infected with bacteria and when incubated in the warmth of a body cavity, they become superb culture media. Bacteria continually invade the host from such a source. Any bacterial toxins elaborated from the culture diffuse directly into the host. Obviously, the first treatment for an infected back in a toxic patient is to remove the source of bacterial inoculum — the gauze pack — immediately upon the recognition of signs of sepsis. Preferably, the pack when used should be removed *before* the infection becomes evident as prophylaxis against septicemia. A Jones pack may also be utilized, particularly if long-term placement of such a pack is for the support of small intestines on extralong mesenteries. Also, occasionally one may wish to use the Jones pack to prevent early intestinal contact with severely irradiated or infected lateral pelvic tissues.

To place a Jones pack in the pelvis, two large Penrose drains are first laid along the lateral pelvic wall and are brought out the perineal incision. A medium weight gum rubber sheet, 36″ × 36″ in size, is cut. This is folded to lie within the pelvis like a sack whose opening is at the perineal wound. Inside this sack, laparotomy gauze is packed tightly to completely fill the pelvis and exert lateral pressure on the pelvis. To hold this pack in, the perineal incision has to be closed partially over it.

When a gauze pack is required in the presence of diffuse capillary or venous bleeding, the packing must be placed under pressure to occlude the bleeding vessels. When the wall of the packed cavity is too yielding to permit intracavitational vascular occlusive pressure, the pack serves no purpose and should not be utilized. The pack actually obstructs drainage, and its only use is for hemostasis and occasionally to support herniating intestines. The rigidity of the pelvic walls permits the proper degree of pressure from the packs. The development of surgical methods to secure primary and complete hemostasis in the pelvis has made the need for packs rare today.

The perineal wound is finally closed in two layers. The subcutaneous tissue is closed with catgut and the skin with silk. When adequate gluteal fat remains, it should be approximated over the coccyx and ischium. This padding makes sitting more comfortable after the wound has healed and the patient has resumed normal activity. A large Penrose drain is used to drain the pelvis through the midpoint of the perineal wound. This perineal closure can be carried out by one or, when available, two members of the surgical team while the other members of the team proceed with the ileal bladder construction.

INTESTINAL INTUBATION

Intestinal obstruction during the postoperative course of patients who have undergone pelvic exenteration has been a hazardous complication. When it occurs it is managed conservatively, if possible, by means of intestinal decompression through a standard long intestinal tube passed through the nose. Reoperation for intestinal obstruction after pelvic exenteration carries an appreciable risk and is to be avoided if possible. In order to avoid the risk of intestinal obstruction and its subsequent complications it has been the practice of one of us (E.M.B.) for years to insert a long intestinal tube from upper jejunum to the terminal ileum for the purpose of decompressing the bowel during the postoperative period and to serve for decompression should obstructive symptoms develop after feeding has started. We do not yet have evidence that use of the tube in this manner decreases the incidence of postoperative obstructive symptoms. However, obstructive symptoms certainly are much easier to manage if the tube is in place, and therefore, reoperation is seldom necessary.

We have found that red rubber tubing ⅛″ by 3/64″ has been most satisfactory. This tubing is procured by the operating room in 50′ lengths and provided to the operating table in segments of 8′, sterilized carefully without kinking or crushing. Small perforations are made by scissors in the distal 3 or 4 feet of tubing, the perforations being approximately 3 inches apart. It is important that the perforations be made carefully and no larger than the lumen of the tube, otherwise the tube would not function distal to the point of the large perforation. Passage of the tube is greatly facilitated by attaching an "introducer" to the distal end with a silk suture. For this purpose we have used a 7 or 8″ segment of ordinary plastic drainage tubing cut with a smooth and beveled distal end. A small opening is made in the upper jejunum about 10 to 12 inches from the ligament of Treitz. If the bowel is as collapsed as it should be after preparation for a pelvic exenteration, introduction of the tubing is greatly facilitated by injecting 300 or 400 cc. of saline solution through the jejunostomy opening. The saline distends the small intestine and acts as a lubricant as the tube is inserted. The plastic introducer with the tube attached is then inserted into the jejunal opening and, with an assistant feeding the tube in, the surgeon can very rapidly manipulate the introducer and carry the tube through the entire small intestine in a relatively short time. It has been our practice to pass the tube through the end-to-end small bowel anastomosis resulting from the ileal segment. The introducer must be removed, and this is done through a small opening in the ileum just proximal to the ileocecal valve where the introducer is delivered and removed and the end of the red rubber tubing is attached to the mucosa of the bowel with a fine catgut stitch in order to prevent it from retracting. The opening resulting from removal of the introducer is closed with catgut and interrupted silk. Additional tubing is then pulled and fed into the small intestine until it smoothly fills all loops of the bowel without crowding or telescoping of the bowel. Kinking of the tube may occur if too much tubing is introduced, and therefore, it is important that this be avoided. The proper amount of tubing will fit the bowel loops smoothly and hold the loops in orderly curves through slight pressure on the antimesenteric bowel wall. After the tubing has been placed in the bowel the jejunal opening is closed over the tubing by the Witzel technique, great care being exercised not to impair the lumen of the bowel at this level. The tube is then brought out through an opening in the abdominal wall at the site considered to be mechanically optimum without producing kinking of the jejunum or of the tube. It has not been our custom to suture the bowel to the parietal peritoneum at the enterostomy site, but this may be done if the surgeon so desires. Five silk sutures would be preferable for this purpose, and it should be done in such a manner that the jejunum is not acutely angulated.

Upon completion of the operation the intubated intestine is placed back into the abdomen in an orderly fashion. It will be found to fit into the pelvis in smooth folds as a "tube plication."

During the postoperative period the tubing is injected forcefully with 2 ounces of normal saline solution every two hours to insure that all perforations are kept open and functioning. Forceful injection cannot be done with a bulb syringe. It is necessary that a piston syringe be used, and the nurses must be instructed regarding the technique of injection. No attempt should be made to withdraw the fluid after injection, for the tube is simply attached to low intermittant suction. This regimen is followed until the patient is taking and tolerating a soft diet, usually five or six days after operation. If the patient has been getting along well, the tube can then be clamped off and simply left in place. At the least sign of abdominal distention or cramping pain the tube can be irrigated and put on suction again. This has been a tremendous advantage compared to the turmoil and delay associated with the insertion of a standard long intestinal tube through the nose.

The tube is not removed until it seems quite certain that the patient will be able to tolerate a normal diet without symptoms. The tube remains in place for a minimum of two weeks postoperatively. After two weeks the holding sutures should separate easily and the site of the jejunostomy should be healed to such an extent that leakage will not occur. The tube is slowly withdrawn over the course of 10 or 15 minutes with rest periods to allow it to retract through the small intestinal loops.

The use of this long intestinal tube has also been found to serve a purpose in the postoperative management of patients who have had surgery for complicated intestinal fistulas or obstruction.

ABDOMINAL CLOSURE

As a preliminary step to closing the abdominal incision, the viscera must be arranged in the abdomen in proper order. Starting with the cecum in the right lower quadrant where it has been brought to a position medial to the ileal segment, the intestines are laid in progressively, starting with the terminal ileum and going from right to left, then back to the right, until the jejunum is reached. If a long tube is used, its proper placement throughout the length of the small intestine is inspected. The end of the tube should have passed through the fresh ileoileal anastomosis performed when the segment of ileum was isolated for the new bladder. It should also pass through the ileocecal valve to lie in the cecum.

A large or long omentum is an anatomical blessing. This great structure should be carefully disentangled from the viscera of the upper abdomen where it usually lies after the packing requisite to obtain pelvic exposure. The omentum is laid smoothly over the small intestines to separate them from the abdominal incision. An omentum of sufficient length may be placed into the deep pelvis, separating the perineal incison from the intestines. The omentum must not be pulled or stretched to fit into the deep pelvis if this risks vascular tear. Occasionally, the omental length can be increased further by insuring that the transverse colon is fully mobilized. The length can also be obtained by detaching the omentum at one side leaving the opposite side attached with blood supply adequate to maintain the vascularity of the entire omentum. The omentum has the remarkable capacity for attaching itself to and assisting in the revascularization and recovery of infected, traumatized and irradiated areas (Spratt, 1960). It protects against the development of adhesions directly between the intestines and irradiated tissue or tissues with no peritoneal coverage.

These preceding steps are easy to bypass in the final moments of the operation. Sponge counts are being made. Preparations are being made for closure of the wound. Fatigue and haste should not supersede these basic steps helpful in protecting the intestines and the peritoneal cavity.

The midline abdominal incision is closed with #28 stainless steel wire swaged on to a large round needle. The suture makes four passes through the abdominal wall — linea alba (right), full thickness of rectus fascia and muscle (left), a full thickness of rectus fascia and muscle (right), and linea alba (left). The sutures are tied just tight enough to approximate the fascia in the midline without producing strangulation necrosis. The skin is approximated with fine silk sutures.

APPLICATION OF STOMAL BAGS AND WOUND DRESSINGS

After the midline abdominal incision is closed, the clamps are removed from the ends of the ileum and colon. The crushed edge of bowel produced by the clamp is opened and the edges of the open ileum and colon are sutured to the skin with interrupted 3–0 silk or chromatized catgut sutures as shown in Figure 8–14. The same procedure is then carried out with end of the colon to approximate the bowel to the skin leaving an everted lip.

The skin about the stomata is dried and sprayed with tincture of benzoin that is allowed to dry for 30 to 60 seconds before the application of the plastic disposable bags to the skin. (Coloplast bags are satisfactory.) The use of benzoin improves the adhesiveness of the plastic bags and helps avoid cutaneous irritations beneath them.

Before the plastic bag is actually applied to a stoma, it is often necessary to enlarge the hole in the center of the adhesive surface. The colostomy, for example, is nearly always greater than the standard 1-inch aperture of most disposable bags. After the hole in the adhesive has been judged adequate, the facing over the adhesive surface is removed and the bag is applied to the prepared skin so that the longitudinal axis of the plastic bag is perpendicular to the midline abdominal incision, and the end of the bag distal from the adhesive surface lies laterally. This position of the bag permits better drainage while the patient is in bed.

When the bag over the stoma of the ileal conduit is in place, a dependent corner of it is cut off and attached to a closed drainage system. This avoids repeated replacement or drainage of urine-filled bags and also facilitates serial measurement of urinary output. When so drained, a properly applied clear plastic bag will stay in place two or three days, after which time a permanent urinary ileostomy bag can be inserted. The principal advantage of the clear plastic bags in the immediate postoperative period is the visual access they allow to the stomata. If after 48 hours the viability of a stoma is not in question, a permanent bag may be applied.

After the stomata are covered, a narrow dry gauze dressing is taped in place over the midline abdominal incision. Dry gauze also is used to cover the perineal incision. Two or three abdominal dressing pads are placed over the perineal gauze and held in place with a T-binder. The transverse arms of this binder are brought around just over the anterior superior iliac spines beneath the urinary and colostomy bags and pinned snuggly to the perpendicular arm of the binder which holds the perineal dressing in place.

HEMIPELVECTOMY

At this point it seems appropriate to report a specific case which considers the actual order of surgery. This case is also unusual in that a hemipelvectomy was performed en bloc with the exenteration. The operative note describes the surgical subroutines added to the standard exenteration to handle an extension of cancer into the musculoskeletal pelvis.

L.D. (62–29997) was first seen at EFSCH in 1962 at the age of 47 with a League of Nations stage III epidermoid carcinoma of the cervix uteri. The cancer recurred after telecobalt and intracavitary curie-

therapy. A pelvic exenteration was performed on July 9, 1964 in continuity with a left hemipelvectomy because of extension of cancer into
the left pelvic wall. That the recurrent cancer involved the pelvic wall
was indeed confirmed by the pathology report. Before surgery this recurrence was associated with intractable sciatica and obstructive
lymphedema. She refused cordotomy for palliation and insisted on the
performance of the radical resection when advised that this approach
offered her the only possible hope for cure.

She was still alive and well in February 1972 at the time of this
writing.

The operative description is published in its entirety to elucidate
an actual case involving nearly all phases of a standard pelvic exenteration with the en bloc performance of a pelvic exenteration.

Preliminary Note

This patient had an advanced stage III cancer of the cervix treated
by radiotherapy in 1962 with a good initial response. Later she developed pain in the distribution of the left sacral plexus and a mass on the
lateral pelvic wall that contained epidermoid cancer on needle
biopsy. She was initially offered a chordotomy to relieve pain but she
declined this in favor of a more radical procedure suggested by Dr.
Sugarbaker for possible total ablation of the recrudescent disease. Dr.
Sugarbaker referred her to the EFSCH for this procedure.

Procedure

Under general endotracheal anesthesia the perineum, abdomen
and skin of the left lower extremity were prepared with a shave, a
Septisol scrub and the application of Betadine and Ioprep solution.
The colon was irrigated with one liter of aqueous Zephiran. The operative field was draped with sterile sheets and towels in the routine
manner with the left lower extremity draped out for free mobility and
with a sandbag beneath the left shoulder to elevate the patient to 45
degrees. An incision was made from one anterior superior iliac spine
to the other, curving inferiorly toward the symphysis pubis. Skin
towels were applied to the margin of the wound before the deep fascia
and the peritoneum were opened. The abdominal cavity was then explored. Both lobes of the liver were normal. The gallbaldder contained several small faceted stones but had no adhesions on it and no
thickening suggestive of inflammation. Both kidneys were of normal

size and contour as was the spleen. The nasogastric tube was placed into the stomach to evacuate air present. No lymph nodes were palpable along the aorta or along either iliac. Except for fibrosis along the internal iliac on the right side, no evidence of residual disease was noted here. Woody induration extended out from the left parametrium and involved the lateral pelvic wall and obstructed the left ureter which was markedly dilated. Operability was ascertained first on the right side, and a standard obturator dissection was performed. The presacral space was entered posteriorly, and the dissection was carried down to the coccyx. The right hypogastric artery and vein were ligated. The lateral pelvic vascular bundles were then clamped between 12" Viet-Harrington clamps, and the bundles were transected and oversewn with continuous figure-of-eight, 0 chromic catgut sutures. The right ureter appeared grossly normal. On the left side the presacral space was entered, and it was ascertained that tumor did not extend across the left sacroiliac joint. Consequently, the common iliac artery and vein on the left side were doubly ligated with 0 silk ligatures and suture ligatures. The markedly dilated left ureter was ligated both proximally and distally. It was transected at the level of the iliac vessels.

This being complete and the bladder being reflected down and away from the retropubic area, the gluteal incision was made through the skin from the iliac crest circumferentially around to the lateral pubis on the left side. This incision was extended down through the gluteus maximus which was elevated posteriorly with the flap to the crest of the ilium and the sacroiliac joint. All musculature along the crest of the ilium was transected down to the upper margin of the sacroiliac joint. Anteriorly, the pubis was transected with a chisel. The vagina and rectum were cut off flush with the perineal floor, and the levator ani muscle on the left side was transected on the left lateral margin of these structures. The levator on the right side was preserved as part of the flap for closure. The areolar tissue of the ischiorectal fossa was cleared away so as to permit access to the lower margin of the sacroiliac joint. The psoas muscle was transected anteriorly. A Gigli saw was passed around the sacroiliac joint and this structure was transected. The proximal sigmoid was cross-clamped between Payr clamps and the sigmoid mesentery was transected between clamps which were suture ligated with 2–0 silk before removal. The specimen was removed from the table. Hemostasis was obtained throughout with cautery coagulation and catgut ligatures. The pelvis was clean of all gross tumor at the completion of the procedure. The stump ends of the sacral plexus showed no gross tumor. The wound margins were then protected with laparotomy gauzes and a section of terminal ileum was taken just proximal to the cecum. The mesentery was divided down to the first arcade. The proximal end was closed with a running 3–0 chromic Connell suture and interrupted silk mattress sutures. An end-to-end, two-layer, interrupted fine silk enteroenterostomy was then effected. The mesenteric defect at the base of the ileal segment was obliterated by suturing the segment and its mesentery to the mesentery of the small bowel and sigmoid, bringing the stump of the segment down to meet the left ureter. An end-to-side, mucosa-to-mucosa ureteroileostomy was performed with an outer layer of interrupted 5–0 arterial silk and an inner layer of interrupted 5–0 chromic catgut. The right ureter was similarly anastomosed. The segment was then brought out through a round incision about 1 inch in diameter in the right lower quadrant and was sutured to the skin with everting 3–0 chromic catgut. The cecum was mobilized and swung medial to the segment. The appendix was removed and the stump ligated and inverted. The remaining mesenteric defect was obliterated with interrupted fine silk sutures. The proximal end of the descending colon was brought out through a similar incison in the left lower quadrant and the mesenteric defect in the left gutter was obliterated with an 0 chromic catgut purse-string suture. After the incision was closed, the colostomy was sutured to the skin similarly to the ileostomy. The abdominal wall was closed in layers with figure-of-eight stainless steel wires to the muscular and fascial layer and continuous 2–0 silk sutures to the skin. Two large Penrose drains with inlying suction catheters were placed through the vaginal orifice, one to the right pelvis and one beneath the flap on the left. The patient tolerated the procedure well and was returned to the postanesthetic recovery room in good condition with a supporting dressing over the wound.

    Fluids: Lactated Ringer's solution, 2000 cc.

             Dextrose in water, 5 per cent, 1150 cc.

             Whole blood, 6 units.

    The pathology specimen (EFSCH pathology #64–1650) confirmed the presence of epidermoid carcinoma infiltrating the soft tissue of the lateral pelvis.

Pathology Report

    Name: L.D.   Age: 49

    Date received in laboratory: 7-9-64   Chart no.: 62-29997

    Gross description: Dr. Spence   Path no.: 64-1650

    The specimen is submitted in one piece and is said to be the result of a left hemipelvectomy and anterior exenteration. The specimen has overall dimensions of 102 cm. superior to inferior aspect and is the left lower extremity in its entirety with the left pelvic bony structure and the entire lower urogenital tract and a segment of rec-

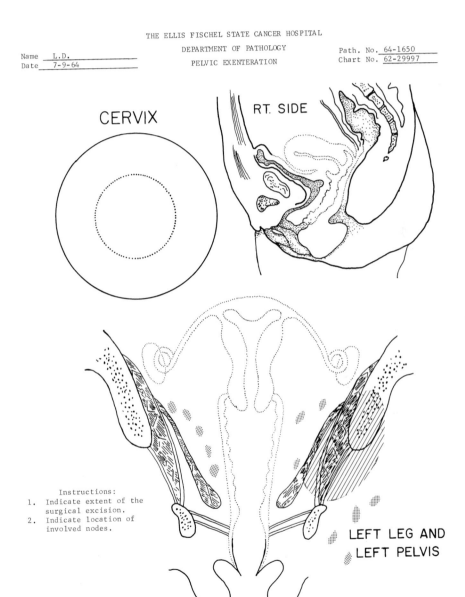

Name L.D.
Date 7-9-64

Path. No. 64-1650
Chart No. 62-29997

CERVIX

RT. SIDE

Instructions:
1. Indicate extent of the surgical excision.
2. Indicate location of involved nodes.

LEFT LEG AND
LEFT PELVIS

Figure 8–16 See *Pathology Report* in text.

tum attached. The vaginal portion which is present measures 10 cm. in circumference at the distal margin of excision and 7 cm. in length. The cervix is markedly stenotic. The vaginal mucosa is gray and thickened but free of ulceration. The cervix has several yellowish areas of exudating lesions 0.5 cm. in diameter visible on the external os. The uterus is atrophic with no palpable lumen. The outside measurement of the uterus is 5×4.5 cm. There is no gross nodularity in the uterus. The right ovary measures $2 \times 1 \times 1$ cm. and is noted to be fibrotic. The right fallopian tube measures 7 cm. in length and is free of nodularity. The left ovary measures $3 \times 1.5 \times 1$ cm. and is fibrotic. The left fallopian tube measures 6 cm. in length and has a palpable contortion 2 cm. from the fimbria. The urethral portion measures 1.5×4 cm. and is noted to be covered with submucosal hemorrhagic spots. The urinary bladder measures 8×11 cm. in inside dimension, and the mucosa was noted to have marked bullous edema. The right ureter measures 8×11 cm. and is noted to have a sharp flexure 3 cm. from the ureterovesical junction. This flexure corresponds to the tumor mass. The mucosa of the ureter is free of tumor involvement. There is a dilated and fibrotic area of the left ureter extending 2.5 cm. distal to the proximal line of surgical excision. There is a length of rectum attached to the specimen measuring 12 cm. in length, 10 cm. in circumference at the proximal line of surgical excision and 6 cm. in circumference at the distal line of surgical excision. There seems to be a moderate amount of fibrosis attaching the upper end of the rectal segment to the other pelvic structures. There is a grossly palpable mass in the iliac fossa between the external iliac artery and the ileum itself. This mass measures 5 cm. in anteroposterior diameter, 7 cm. in superoinferior dimension and 4 cm. in lateral dimension. This mass was adherent to the iliac process but could be dissected easily from it. There is no gross involvement of the ileum by this mass. The mass extended to within 1 cm. of the sacral iliac articulation and extends to within 3 cm. of the line of surgical separation of the iliac bone itself. The mass extends to the anterior margin of the greater foramen and to within 8 cm. of the symphysis pubis. The external iliac artery was encroached upon by this tumor mass, distorting its course, but there is no gross involvement of the endothelial lining. The external iliac vein was also distorted by this tumor mass and there is a gray-red organizing thrombus at the point of deflection. A portion of this thrombus is intraluminal, and a portion of the thrombus is intramural. The obturator and femoral nerves are both encroached upon by this mass, but it is difficult to ascertain grossly their involvement. The rest of the extremity appears grossly normal.

Sections were taken as follows:

(A)	tumor	(I)	colon
(B)	appendix	(J)	bladder

(C) vagina
(D) cervix
(E) uterus
(F) right ovary and oviduct
(G) left ovary and oviduct
(H) rectum

(K) urethra
(L) right ureter
(M) left ureter
(N) right lymph nodes
(O) left lymph nodes
(P) inguinal lymph nodes

Addendum: The specimen was reexamined, and some additional sections were taken from the area in which the tumor appeared to be in close contact with some of the pelvic vessels. Sections were taken as follows:

(Q) vein and tumor
(R) tumor including vessels and left ureter
(S) uterus
(T) urinary bladder

Microscopic Description

This is a mid-differentiated epidermoid carcinoma which infiltrates, as is grossly described, the soft tissue of the pelvis, left side, invading numerous structures including midsize veins and arteries, nerves, and is close to the serosa of the left ureter. In some of the vessels, although no tumor is seen extending into the lumen, the wall has been questionably involved by the tumor; in some areas this is represented by irregular nests of closely packed midsize cells which are formed in irregular lobules separated by fibrohyalinized tissue. There is fibroblastic proliferation, and in some vessels there are numerous subendothelial vacuoles seen as an effect of irradiation. No remnants of tumor were present in the section from the cervix and sections from the body of the uterus as from the ovaries show atrophy and fibrosis. No abnormal changes are seen in the sections from the colon. Sections from the bladder show chronic inflammation of the mucosa, but no actual tumor infiltration is observed. A section of the tumor involving the neighboring tip of the sacrum is decalcified, and after this procedure is completed an additional report will be issued. Twelve lymph nodes were dissected, and no metastases were observed. In summary, this is a mid-differentiated epidermoid carcinoma, metastatic from the cervix which infiltrates numerous structures in the soft tissue of the pelvis. No recurrent tumor was found in the cervix.

Microscopic Diagnoses

Soft tissue, pelvis (pelvic exenteration in continuity with hemipelvectomy)—metastatic mid-differentiated epidermoid carcinoma with vascular infiltration, primary Cervix, see above description.

Uterus—atrophy
            —irradiation effect
Ovaries and tubes—atrophy
Urinary bladder, terminal ureters—chronic inflammation
Colon, large intestine, sigmoid—chronic inflammation
Lymph nodes, pelvis—hyperplasia, 12/12
Appendix, (appendectomy)—appendix

Note: The leg has been used for dissecting purposes; after this procedure is completed, a report will be issued (no additional diagnoses C.P.M./6-2-65).

REFERENCES

Cook, G. B., and Watson, F. R.: SURTRAN, Linear graphing of surgical decisions and activities. J. Surg. Res., 9:361, 1969.

Long, R. T. L., Grummon, R. A., Spratt, J. S., Jr., and Perez-Mesa, C.: Carcinoma of the urinary bladder (comparison with radical, simple and partial cystectomy and intravesical formalin). Cancer, 29:98, 1972.

Spratt, J. S., Jr., Donegan, W. L., and Rapp, M.: Positioning and some variations in surgical technique used for combined inguinal perineal and abdominal cancer surgery. Am. J. Obstet. Gynecol., 99:417, 1967.

Spratt, J. S., Jr., Heinbecker, P., and Saltzstein, S.: The influence of succinyl-sulfathiazole (sulfasuxidine-Merck) upon the response of canine small intestine to irradiation. Cancer, 14:862, 1960.

Spratt, J. S., Jr., Shieber, W., and Dillard, B. M.: Anatomy and Surgical Technique of Groin Dissection. Saint Louis, The C. V. Mosby Co., 1965.

Chapter Nine

POSTOPERATIVE CARE

The postoperative care of patients having undergone pelvic exenteration follows the pattern of that for any major abdominal operation. In addition, special emphasis must be placed on several areas of observation and care because of the extended nature of the operation. The following discussion of the facets of postoperative care is presented in order of relative and chronological importance. Beyond these special comments, the guidelines contained in the *Manual of Preoperative and Postoperative Care,* American College of Surgeons, are also relevant.

PULMONARY FUNCTION

The patient will have had prolonged anesthesia, multiple blood transfusions, and large amounts of water and electrolyte solutions. The problem will be compounded if the patient has demonstrated any evidence of preoperative pulmonary functional impairment. Full advantage should be taken of modern methods of estimating adequacy of ventilation. Incipient respiratory failure may be very difficult to diagnose without frequent measurements of tidal volume, pulmonary mechanics and arterial blood gases. If there is any question about the adequacy of respiratory function, the patient should be placed in an intensive care unit where the necessary monitoring is easily available. The endotracheal tube should not be removed until the respiratory status appears to be stabilized. There should be no hesitation in keeping the patient on artificial ventilation for 24 hours, 48 hours or longer if necessary. Because of the massive blood and fluid replacements that may have been necessary, the patient should be observed critically for evidence of pulmonary vascular congestion or pulmonary edema.

After the acute postoperative phase has passed, the patient will need aggressive care to promote the elimination of pulmonary secretions and to prevent the development of hypostatic congestion and resultant infection. It is our custom to use broad-spectrum antibiotic coverage during the immediate postoperative period.

RESTORATION OF BLOOD VOLUME

During the course of the operation the patient will have had blood replacement based upon measured and estimated blood loss. Assuming the patient is relatively normovolemic at the termination of surgery, it should be realized that the loss of red blood cells and plasma into the operative area, the wound and the pelvic defect will be continuous over the next several days even without the obvious active bleeding. All parameters of blood volume and red blood cell measurement will be necessary for accurate appraisal, including the standard values of central venous pressure, urinary output, hemoglobin, hematocrit, pulse and arterial pressure. It is usual for the patient to require an additional unit of blood at some time during the evening or night of the day of the operation. The need for more blood (one or two units) becomes apparent after the hemodynamic factors have stabilized after 48 to 72 hours. If active bleeding has been present in the immediate postoperative period, blood replacement will be indicated volume for volume insofar as this can be estimated. It becomes a matter of surgical judgment when active bleeding should be treated by simple replacement or by a return to the operating room for control.

WATER AND ELECTROLYTE BALANCE

During the course of a standard uncomplicated pelvic exenteration, the patient will have been on the operating table at least three or four hours and will have received three or four units of whole blood and 2000 or 3000 ml. water and electrolyte solution. In addition to the standard vital signs, the central venous pressure and evidence of continued urinary output during the course of the operation are of great importance in determining whether replacement of blood volume, water and electrolytes has been adequate. After the ureters have been cut it is possible to observe urinary secretion from the proximal cut end, though this is not a practical means of estimating volume output. After the ureters are anastomosed to the ileal segment, the secretion of urine should be observable through the segment stoma and should be measurable upon completion of the operation. The sequestration and loss of extracellular fluid into the operative area and from the denuded surfaces is excessive and continuous for many hours after the operation is completed. As in the treatment of burns, it has been found that the most satisfactory replacement solution has been a balanced crystalloid solution (Ringer's lactate). During the immediate postoperative period the need for this type of replacement must be balanced with the need for whole blood and is best monitored by the central venous pressure and hourly urinary output. The average patient is almost certain to require 3000 to 4000 ml. crystalloid solution, with the majority of this being balanced salt. Subsequent volume and ratio of salt solution to water can be monitored by blood electrolyte and pH determinations.

URINARY OUTPUT

The preceding paragraphs indicate the importance of adequate replacement therapy in the maintenance of secretory renal function. Ideally, a urinary output of 30 to 50 ml. per hour should be maintained from the time of the operation. An appreciable drop in urine output is a good indication of inadequate replacement therapy. We find hypovolemia to be the most frequent cause of diminished or absent urinary flow in the early postoperative period. The differential diagnosis between hypovolemia and other causes of oliguria or anuria may be somewhat difficult. First, fluid replacement during and subsequent to the operation should be compared with estimated requirements in order to be sure that the patient hasn't been undertreated. Any deficit should be corrected. If this does not lead to urinary secretion, a short trial of loading the kidneys plus the use of a diuretic will frequently precipitate urine flow. This must be done with circumspection and careful attention to the central venous pressure. If correction of hypovolemia plus a trial by loading and a diuretic do not produce a urine flow, the other causes for anuria must be considered.

Acute Tubular Necrosis

If, in addition to the prolonged operation, the patient has had a period of shock requiring multiple blood transfusions, it is quite possi-

ble for renal damage to have occurred. It would be unusual for immediate anuria to be due to acute tubular necrosis, since the usual
clinical course is an initial urinary output which steadily declines over
the following 24 to 48 hours. The diagnosis of acute tubular necrosis
should not be entertained until underhydration and other causes of
anuria have been ruled out. Once the diagnosis is made, the standard
treatment is put into effect.

Bilateral Ureteral Obstruction

When the operation of urinary diversion to an ileal segment is
done by a competent surgeon, the chance of bilateral ureteral obstruction is less than 1 per cent. There is a chance that one ureter will be
completely and permanently obstructed. However, one functional
kidney is enough to carry the patient through the postoperative
period, and the obstructed ureter is usually not recognized until intravenous pyelograms are made before the patient is discharged from
the hospital. Obstruction of the external ileal stoma is a rare complication. During a period of decreased urinary output, a mucus plug may
form in the stoma and may obstruct the lumen for a time. The condition of the external stoma and its patency should be one of the first
things to determine when the urinary output is unsatisfactory. A small
catheter passed into the stoma will demonstrate a retention of urine, if
present. The adequacy of the opening through the abdominal wall
would have been determined at the time of the operation. Usually a
curved Kelly clamp passed gently into the segment and spread will
verify adequacy of this opening. The color of the visible portion of the
external stoma is important to note, since evidence of necrosis may
mean that the entire segment is necrotic.

Extravasation

A leak of one or both ureterointestinal anastomoses is, of course,
possible. The urine may escape into the pelvis and out the pelvic
drain site or into the peritoneal cavity. An x-ray of the ileal segment
after the injection of opaque solution (a retrograde ileogram) will demonstrate whether or not a leak is present. It may also be helpful in
demonstrating reflux through the ureters which would be a strong indication that obstruction of the anastomoses is not present. While the
patient is having these x-ray studies, intravenous pyelograms might be
helpful. The demonstration of a bilateral excretory shadow without

any evidence of extravasation is a good indication that no leak is present and that the patient does not have acute tubular necrosis.

Edema of Ureterointestinal Anastomosis

After ruling out the various possible causes of oliguria and anuria listed above, it is our policy to "sit tight" for 48 to 72 hours with the expectation that urine will eventually come through. We are quite certain that there is such a thing as temporary and partial mechanical or functional obstruction of the ureteral anastomoses. Relatively frequently we have seen patients who put out very little or no urine for varying periods of time in the immediate postoperative period, followed by the sudden appearance of urine which from that time on is secreted in normal amounts. We postulate that the temporary obstruction due to edema resolved and the pressure of urinary excretion became enough to cause the anastomoses to start functioning.

From the foregoing discussion, it is evident that reoperation for decreased or absent urinary output can usually be avoided. The positive indications for early reoperation are necrosis or retraction of the ileal segment and disruption of one or both ureteral intestinal anastomoses with demostration of a leak. Bilateral ureteral obstruction with complete anuria is extremely unlikely in our experience, and there is no great hurry in reoperating if it is suspected. All other possible causes of anuria should be ruled out as completely as possible. It can be disastrous to reoperate for ureteral obstruction and find that the anuria is due to some other cause. The status of the renal collection system assayed by intravenous pyelography during an eight-year period after the performance of an ileal bladder is shown in Figures 8–4 to 8–15.

ANTIBIOTIC THERAPY

There is good evidence that broad-spectrum antibiotic coverage immediately preoperatively and for three to five days after the operation has merit in preventing postoperative infections and pneumonitis. The operation of pelvic exenteration is unavoidably contaminated. Prophylactic antibiotic therapy may help to insure the integrity of anastomoses, suture lines and the viability of irradiated bowel with marginal blood supply. If definite infection appears in the wound, urine or in the pelvic defect, it is important that the causative organism and its sensitivities be determined as rapidly as possible in order that specific antibiotic therapy may be instituted.

INCOMPATIBILITY OF DRUGS FOR INTRAVENOUS ADMINISTRATION

Patients undergoing pelvic exenteration may be on intravenous fluids, electrolytes and other drugs for several days. A factor in postoperative fluid and drug administration that is frequently overlooked and that has been incompletely studied, is the incompatibility of drugs used for intravenous administration. The mixtures in intravenous fluids may include varying electrolyte composition, pH and a host of drugs including antibiotics, pressor amines, vitamins and numerous other agents. Many of these agents are physically or chemically incompatible with one another, leading to precipitation, inactivation and change in effects. Certain warning signs of incompatibility among mixtures include color change, haze, effervescence and precipitation.

Effects of pH. Changes in pH when two drugs are mixed may affect the stability of one or both agents. The inactivation of potassium penicillin G by ascorbic acid is an example of the effects of such changes. Since most tetracycline hydrochloride solutions for intravenous administration contain ascorbic acid as a buffering agent, the same effect occurs when such a solution is mixed with a solution of potassium penicillin G.

Tetracycline hydrochloride alone has an acid pH and degrades penicillin, but the ascorbic acid lowers the pH of the final solution to such an extent that the penicillin may be almost completely inactivated if the mixture remains at room temperature for many hours (Im). Lactate solution and lactated Ringer's injection (U.S.P.) may have pH values inimical to the stability of some of the drugs which are added to them. When such solutions are used care should be taken to see that the optimum pH of the drug to be administered is maintained.

While physical evidence of incompatibility does not necessarily mean therapeutic inactivation (buffers or other additives may be incompatible rather than the drugs themselves), mixtures which show evidence of physical incompatibility should be discarded. The fact that a given combination of drugs is not designated *incompatible* in Table 6–1 (see Chap. Six) does not imply that the combination is *compatible;* data on compatibility are not available for most mixtures of specific agents.

Since changes in pH and other factors can cause deterioration of drugs when they are mixed in solutions, unless it is known that drugs are compatible, they should be administered separately. Separate administration offers the further advantage of greater control over the rate of administration of each drug.

For further information on incompatibility of drugs see the package brochures of the drugs which occasionally contain information on incompatibilities. Also, see Meisler, J. M., and Skolaut, M. W.: Extemporaneous sterile compounding of intravenous additives. Am. J. Hosp. Pharm., 23:557, 1966; Dunworth, R. D., and Kenna, F. R.: Am. J. Hosp. Pharm., 22:190, 1965. Table 6–1 (see Chap. Six) is based on these sources and on information from the *Medical Letter on Drugs and Therapeutics*, most of the major pharmaceutical manufacturers and on other similar sources.

MOBILIZATION OF THE PATIENT

Early ambulation is difficult to put into practice with the exenteration patient because of awkwardness occasioned by various tubes, appliances and dressings. For the patients with a huge perineal wound, the discomfort caused by getting up or sitting further precludes against early mobilization. Accordingly, efforts must be doubled to use all measures possible to prevent venous thrombosis. These measures include elastic stockings or bandages, leg exercises and frequent turning of the patient. As with all other major surgical cases, it is important that the exenteration patients be mobilized as rapidly as possible.

CARE OF ILEOSTOMY STOMA

In order to measure urinary output, the patient will have had some type of temporary glued-on appliance placed in the operating room. This will usually be a transparent plastic bag to which a drainage tube is connected. The transparency allows inspection of the ileostomy stoma without removing the bag. As soon as it is apparent that the ileostomy stoma is receiving an adequate blood supply and is functioning satisfactorily, the temporary bag may be replaced by one of the permanent types. There are numerous brands of ileostomy bags which have been adapted for the urinary ileostomy by the insertion of a valve mechanism for drainage. It is not necessary that the bag stoma fit the ileostomy stoma as exactly as is desirable with a fecal ileostomy. It is of the greatest importance that the bag be applied expertly, preferably by someone who has had experience in its use. It is also very important that it be observed closely by an experienced individual in order that complications referable to the bag can be recognized early and appropriately treated. In hospitals with an adequate volume of colonic and ileal stomata, a stomal therapist can be a very great help. In the absence of a stomal therapist, it becomes the responsibility of the operating surgeon to see that the problems referable to the urinary ileostomy are promptly recognized and solved. If care is not taken in the management of the ileostomy, it can be very troublesome. The skin can become excoriated, and the bag may not stick; the patient will be constantly wet with urine with the result that the patient, the surgeon and the entire nursing staff embark on a several days' ordeal that should have been prevented. It may become necessary to leave the bag off entirely and to let the urine drain into bulky dressings while the skin heals, after which another attempt at the bag application is made.

There are several appliances on the market that are specifically devised for urinary ileostomies. They consist basically of a flat bag made of rubber or plastic material attached to a flange that fits over the ileostomy stoma. They are attached to the skin either by a double-faced adhesive or by surgical cement. The size and shape of the aperture through the flange can be tailored and custom-made to fit the type of ileostomy stoma. However, it is our practice to keep a supply of bags with apertures of 1¼ inch in width. This size is satisfactory for the average uncomplicated case. An occasional patient will develop an inflammatory, condylomatous reaction in the skin immediately around the ileostomy stoma. This reaction appears to be due to continuous wetness from urine, and it can only be alleviated by a bag which fits the stoma exactly. It may be necessary eventually to review the ileostomy stoma before a perfect fit can be obtained. The patient should be taught to apply the bag himself as rapidly as his postoperative condition permits. It is very necessary that he be capable and feel competent in his ability to manage the bag before discharge from the hospital. A sample of the type of instructions that are supplied to the patient at the time of his discharge is given in Appendix 3.

ALIMENTATION

Patients having undergone pelvic exenteration are prone to have a rather prolonged period of intestinal ileus. They are kept on decompression either through a nasogastric or gastrostomy tube until it is quite certain that effective peristalsis is reestablished and the colostomy is functioning. Because of the eviscerated pelvis and the resultant dislocation of the small intestine, there is a relatively high incidence of postoperative intestinal obstruction. For this reason, it is most important to start feedings very carefully; the patient must not be allowed to become markedly distended if his gastrointestinal tract is not yet functionally adequate. Rarely are oral feedings started before the fifth postoperative day. Mechanical small bowel obstruction should be recognized early and promptly treated by the use of a long intestinal tube in the hope that the obstruction will be relieved and that reoperation may not be necessary.

If a long intestinal tube has been inserted through the jejunum at the time of the operation, the dangers of postoperative ileus and obstruction are obviated to a great degree. It is the practice to keep these long tubes irrigated and on suction for three or four days after feedings are started. When the patient is able to take a soft diet without symptoms, the tube is simply clamped off. If ileus, cramping pain or bowel distention occur at any time subsequently, the tube is irrigated and put on suction. The chance of intestinal obstruction requiring reoperation is reduced by the use of a long tube in this manner.

CARE OF COLOSTOMY

Colostomy care in the postoperative period of exenteration patients does not differ greatly from that of any other patient with a left-sided colostomy. Effective colonic function is likely to be delayed somewhat longer, partly as a result of the relatively prolonged period of the small intestinal ileus. Ordinarily, a small enema is given on the third or fourth postoperative day for the purpose of stimulating peristalsis in the distal colonic segment. Following this, daily colonic irrigations are given with gradually increasing amounts of irrigating fluid up to a 1000 or 1500 ml. Tap water is the standard irrigating fluid, although isotonic salt solution may be advisable if there is an appreciable retention of the irrigating fluid over several days. The patient with a normal postoperative course should have developed effective peristalsis and adequate colostomy function by the fifth or sixth postoperative day. It is inadvisable to start oral feeding until this time.

The patient is made acquainted with the colostomy as soon as possible and is encouraged to help with the irrigation just as quickly as this seems practical. By the end of the first week after the operation, the patient should be participating actively in the irrigation ritual. An ideal patient with an uncomplicated postoperative course should be capable of taking care of both the ileostomy appliance and the colostomy irrigation by the end of the second postoperative week. He cannot accomplish this without active and informed help and assistance, however. To slough the job off onto inexperienced members of the nursing staff or resident staff can only lead to delayed progress, excoriation of skin, a misbehaving colostomy, and a discouraged and depressed patient. A trained stomal therapist can be an invaluable aid to the patient during this period. In the absence of trained and expert assistants, it is the surgeon's responsibility to see that the stomal problems are solved and that the nursing staff and the house staff are properly instructed. If the surgeon is not willing to deal with the solution of these problems or is unwilling to give the time necessary to instruct the patient adequately, he should not perform this type of surgery. The instructions supplied to colostomy patients on discharge from the Ellis Fischel State Cancer Hospital are given in Appendix 4.

RECTAL FUNCTION AFTER ANTERIOR EXENTERATION

The anterior rectal wall is subjected to varying amounts of surgical trauma during the course of anterior exenteration. It is wise for the surgeon to have determined not only that there is no perforation of the rectal wall but also that there is no area of near perforation which may contribute to a rectovaginal or rectopelvic fistula in the postoperative period. This can be done during the course of the operation by ballooning the rectum with normal saline after the exenteration has been completed. Such a procedure may demonstrate areas in the anterior rectal wall in which the muscularis has been damaged to such an extent that nothing but mucosa is left intact. Such areas should be carefully repaired and reinforced by pulling the muscularis together over them, preferably with fine catgut.

Spontaneous bowel movements may be very slow in developing. Because of the removal of the pelvic peritoneum and the anterior viscera, the patient is unable to exert any pressure on the rectum to aid in the expulsion of feces. For this reason, it is necessary to give enemas to promote evacuation. This should be done with great care in the postoperative period. The first enema is rarely given before the fifth postoperative day. The preferred enema is 90 cc. of equal parts of warm mineral oil, glycerin and water. It is given primarily as a stimulant for rectal peristalsis. The anterior rectal wall could easily be perforated by the too energetic insertion of a large catheter or colon tube. Practically normal rectal function may be expected to develop eventually. Until this time, the patient may have to rely on mild laxatives and rectal irrigation in order to promote satisfactory evacuation.

CARE OF RESIDUAL PELVIC DEFECT AND ABDOMINAL WOUNDS

After total pelvic exenteration, the residual pelvic defect will seldom be obliterated completely before the patient is ready for discharge from the hospital. In roughly half the cases, the defect will be so small that rapid healing may be anticipated. Obliteration of the defect results from descent of the small intestine into the pelvis and by growth of granulation tissue and contracture of whatever defect is

left. The remaining 50 per cent of the patients may have a large residual defect by the time they leave the hospital. It is important that the
extent of this defect be appreciated as early as possible. Occasionally,
drainage of the pelvic defect at the time of operation may not be adequate to dispose of the small amount of bleeding that may be present
when the operation is completed. In such a case, the defect may fill up
with blood which forms a large clot. When such a clot forms, it is certain eventually to become infected and the sooner it is recognized the
better. A good practice is to remove the perineal drain on the sixth or
seventh postoperative day and to explore the residual defect with a
sterile, gloved index finger. If a large empty cavity is encountered, it
becomes obvious that the perineal drain site will have to kept open for
adequate drainage until healing occurs by secondary intention. If a
large clot is encountered, it is equally obvious that the sooner it is
evacuated, the sooner normal healing will progress. Clinically, the
presence of a large clot becoming infected may become evident six to
eight days from the time of operation when the temperature takes an
unexplained rise. This would usually be followed by the development
of foul-smelling drainage through the perineal drain site. The presence of the clot, infected or otherwise, should be detected as early as
possible, and its expulsion encouraged by daily saline irrigations.
Mobilizing the patient to the sitting position will frequently promote
the expulsion of the clot. The use of half-strength hydrogen peroxide
solution as an irrigating agent has much in its favor, since it tends to
break up clots and debride the defect. However, hydrogen peroxide
must not be used unless it is absolutely certain that the wound is old
enough so that the loops of intestine have walled off the free peritoneal cavity and unless the perineal opening to the outside is adequate enough to prevent the accumulation of pressure. We have not
found it necessary to resort to irrigation with proteolytic enzymes.
When the patient with a residual pelvic defect is ready to go home, it
is important that arrangements be made for his close follow-up either
as an outpatient by the surgeon himself or by a responsible local
physician who understands the importance of keeping the perineal
drain site open and the perineal wound clean. Some of the larger
defects may require several months before healing completely. If this
aspect of postoperative care is neglected, the perineal drain site may
close over a residual wound cavity and an abscess will form in the
empty space. When this happens, the walls of the defect become rigid,
and it may take even longer for healing to occur.

REHABILITATION

The abdominal wound care is no different from that provided for
similar abdominal incisions. Careful fascia-to-fascia and skin-to-skin

approximation of the incision without tension and in the presence of good hemostasis is even more important when the incision extends through an irradiated region. Also, the skin sutures are left in several days longer than is usually the practice, since healing of irradiated tissue proceeds at a slower rate and wound separation infection and tissue necrosis are more serious (Spratt).

Rehabilitation of the patient should have started before the operation was done. When it was first discussed, it should have been explained that returning to an active life and normal activity could be anticipated. After the operation, early instruction of the patient regarding care of the altered excretory functions should be accompanied by daily encouragement and moral support. It takes mental fortitude and determination for the patient to survive the magnitude of the operation and the alterations in her life that it entails. She will require support and understanding. At the same time, a very firm hand may have to be used for some patients who may develop a reaction of self-pity and chronic invalidism. These patients can be recognized without too much difficulty and must be handled firmly but kindly.

An unfortunate part of the problem of rehabilitation resides in the relatively young female cured of her cancer and physically well but sexually incapacitated. It is for this type of patient that vaginal reconstructive procedures have been attempted in recent years. These procedures add to the magnitude and complications of the operation and are not always functionally successful. In the absence of a functional vaginal reconstruction, there is not much that can be done about the situation. Undoubtedly, some of the young husbands have wandered and a few instances are known in which the husband left and did not return. However, most of the husbands who are sexually active enough for this to have presented a problem have stood by their wives and have held their home together. We are not unmindful of this undesirable effect of the operation. However, we have been absorbed by the problems of curing the patient of cancer and have not made a detailed study of the effects of sexual incapacitation.

Some of the subroutines of exenterative pelvic surgery, such as a simultaneous hemipelvectomy, create special problems in rehabilitation and prosthetic design, requiring the consultation of specialists in rehabilitation early in the postoperative period when special problems are anticipated.

REFERENCES

Im, S., and Latiolais, C. J.: Physico-chemical incompatibilities of parenteral admixtures — penicillin and tetracyclines. Am. J. Hosp. Pharm., 23:333, 1966.
Spratt, J. S., Jr., and Sala, J. M.: The healing of wounds within irradiated tissue. Mo. Med., 59:409, 1962.

Chapter Ten

POSTOPERATIVE AND LATE COMPLICATIONS ATTRIBUTABLE TO THE PROCEDURE OF PELVIC EXENTERATION

Operative mortality for pelvic exenteration has reached a rate of 10 per cent or less as the technique of the operation has improved, as operative time has decreased and as the volume of required blood replacement has declined incident to less operative blood loss and the liberal use of Ringer's solution with lactate during the operation (Tables 10–1 and 10–2). Ninety patients treated in the Barnes Hospital by exenteration of the pelvic organs during the five-year period from 1960 to 1965 sustained a hospital mortality of 7 per cent (six patients). One decade earlier (1950–1954) 10 of 75 (14 per cent) died. Depsite the improvement in immediate hospital mortality, the morbidity of pelvic exenteration is high (Kiselow) (Tables 10–3 and 10–4).

Serious postoperative complications occurred among 92 of the 207 women treated by pelvic exenteration for recurrent postirradiational carcinoma of the cervix. Sixteen of the 92 died of their complications. Sepsis, most often incident to infection arising in the pelvic defect, occurred in 19 per cent of the patients. Intestinal obstruction also was a serious postoperative problem. Of 24 patients developing the signs of postoperative intestinal obstruction, 9 required reopera-

Table 10–1 Operative Mortality Rates Following Pelvic
Exenteration for Carcinoma of the Cervix by Five-Year Intervals[*]

INTERVAL	NUMBER OF PATIENTS	NUMBER OF OPERATIVE DEATHS	OPERATIVE MORTALITY RATE (%)
1950–1954	75	10	13.4
1955–1959	78	5	6.4
1960–1965	54	1	1.8
Total	207	16	7.8

[*]From Kiselow, M., Butcher, H. R., Jr., and Bricker, E. M.: Results of the radical surgical treatment of advanced pelvic cancer: a fifteen-year study. Ann. Surg., *166*:428, 1967.

tion. Five of these patients died, usually of persistent partial obstruction and enteroperineal fistula.

Except for sepsis and intestinal obstruction, the other complications listed in Table 10–3 have become rare. For example, bleeding as a course of postoperative death has not occurred since 1956. Ureteral obstruction or necrosis requiring operative revision, convulsions, thrombosis of the external iliac artery and acoustic nerve damage (from neomycin) have not been seen in the past decade.

The continual occurrence of complications months and years after exenteration of the pelvic organs makes it essential that surgeons performing the operation be willing to assume long-term responsibility for these patients. Serious illness incident to the operation occurred in 75 of 191 patients who survived the operation (Table 10–4). As in the immediate postoperative period, small intestinal obstruction and related enteroperineal fistulas remain serious late complications. Nine of 14 perineal fistulas were in the small intestine; five were incident to coloanal anastomoses. Late complications incident to the ileal conduit have been infrequent. Only three patients required late

Table 10–2 Operative Mortality Rates Following
Pelvic Exenteration for All Lesions[*]

INTERVAL	NUMBER OF PATIENTS	NUMBER OF OPERATIVE DEATHS	OPERATIVE MORTALITY RATE %)
1950–1960	222	26	12
1960–1965	90	6	7
Total	312	32	10

[*]From Kiselow, M., Butcher, H. R., Jr., and Bricker, E. M.: Results of the radical surgical treatment of advanced pelvic cancer: a fifteen-year study. Ann. Surg., *166*:428, 1967.

Table 10–3 Postoperative Complications in 92 of 207 Women
After Pelvic Exenteration for Persistent Carcinoma of the Cervix*

POSTOPERATIVE COMPLICATION	NUMBER OF PATIENTS HAVING EACH COMPLICATION		NUMBER OF PATIENTS DYING POSTOPERATIVELY
1. Intestinal obstruction		24	6
Treated by laparotomy	9		5
Treated without laparotomy	15		1
2. Hemorrhage		8	3
3. Ileal stoma separation		4	1
4. Colostomy stoma separation		2	
5. Ureteral obstruction or necrosis		3	1
6. Fecal or urinary fistula		6	
7. Acute pyelonephritis		8	1
8. Postoperative psychosis		4	1
9. Wound infection, pelvic abscess, peritonitis		39	
10. Convulsions		5	1
11. Thrombosis of iliac artery		1	
12. Thrombophlebitis		8	
13. Heart failure		2	1
14. Cerebrovascular accident		1	1
15. Acoustic nerve damage		2	
16. Miscellaneous (tracheostomy, atelectasis, osteitis, pubis, parotitis)		6	
Total complications		123	16

Note: 115 patients had no complications; 67 had one complication; and 25 had more than one complication.
*From Kiselow, M., Butcher, H. R., Jr., and Bricker, E. M.: Results of the radical surgical treatment of advanced pelvic cancer: a fifteen-year study. Ann. Surg., *166*:428, 1967.

revision of the ileal bladder for progressive hydronephrosis. Twelve others had bouts of acute pyelonephritis controlled with antibiotics (usually tetracycline).

Incisional hernias are an occasional late complication for all types of abdominal surgery. The abdominal and parastomal hernias would have the standard indications for repair not meriting special consideration in this book. They must be quite infrequent, however, since only a few cases are known to exist.

Of more frequent occurrence is the occasional hernia through the perineal wound. This can occur only in patients with an exceptionally long mesentery. Most mesenteries are too short to permit perineal herniation. Occasionally, a mesentery is so long as to permit immediate or early postoperative herniation before the perineal wound has healed. When this situation is recognized at the completion of the exenteration, the placement of a Jones pack in the perineal wound is

Table 10–4   Complications in 75 of 191 Women Who Left the Hospital After Having Had Pelvic Exenteration for Carcinoma of the Cervix*

LATE COMPLICATION		NUMBER OF PATIENTS HAVING EACH COMPLICATION
1. Intestinal obstruction		12
Operation	10	
Tube only	2	
2. Progressive hydronephrosis requiring ileal bladder revision		3
3. Enteroperineal fistula		9
Due to recurrent carcinoma	2	
Without recurrent carcinoma	7	
4. Rectoperineal fistula		5†
Due to recurrent carcinoma	1	
Without recurrent carcinoma	4	
5. Pyelonephritis		12
6. Ileal stoma revision		14
7. Colostomy revision		16
8. Perineal sinus or abscess		7
9. Perineal hernia		4
10. Renal calculus		2
11. Serum hepatitis		1
12. Thrombophlebitis		1
13. Incisional hernia		1
14. Osteitis pubis		1
Total complications‡		88

Note: 116 patients had no further complications referable to the operation.

*From Kiselow, M., Butcher, H. R., Jr., and Bricker, E. M.: Results of the radical surgical treatment of advanced pelvic cancer: a fifteen-year study. Ann. Surg., *166*:428, 1967.

†Rectoperineal fistulas occurred in five of nine women having coloanal anastomoses.

‡Complications incident to recurrent cancer not included except as noted (items 3 and 4).

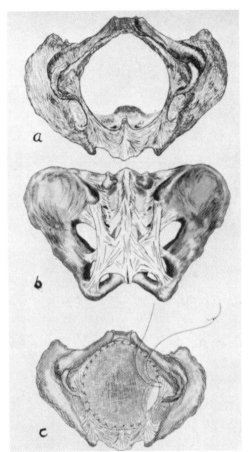

Figure 10–1 Schematic composition of the bony and ligamentous structures of the pelvis: a, View from pelvic outlet; b, posterior view; c, suturing of a prosthetic device to the pelvic ligaments. (From Ego-Aguirre, E., Spratt, J. S., Jr., Butcher, H. R., Jr., and Bricker, E. M.: Repair of perineal hernias developing subsequent to pelvic exenteration. Ann. Surg., *159*:66, 1964.)

necessary to support the intestines until they have become adherent to lateral pelvis. The pack is removed slowly over a number of days.

When the perineal hernia develops months to years after the operation, the hernias can become quite large and symptomatic. When reviewed in 1964 by Ego-Aguirre et al. perineal hernias had developed in 9 of 80 long-term survivors (11.2 per cent). Repair of these hernias is indicated when they produce symptoms from pain or their size is so great as to risk pressure necrosis of the intestine from assuming a sitting position. The technique for repairing the defect is shown in Figures 10–1 to 10–4.

In repairing these hernias great care must be exercised to avoid intestinal injury. Mechanical and antibiotic preparation of the intestine and the passage of a Miller-Abbott tube throughout the intestine must both be accomplished in the preoperative period. All three

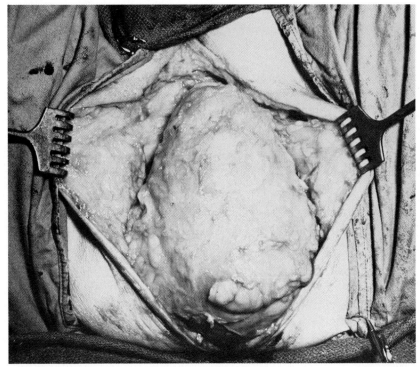

Figure 10–2 Large hernial sac as presented after subcutaneous elevation of skin flaps. (From Ego-Aguirre, E., Spratt, J. S., Jr., Butcher, H. R., Jr., and Bricker, E. M.: Repair of perineal hernias developing subsequent to pelvic exenteration. Ann. Surg., *159*:66, 1964.)

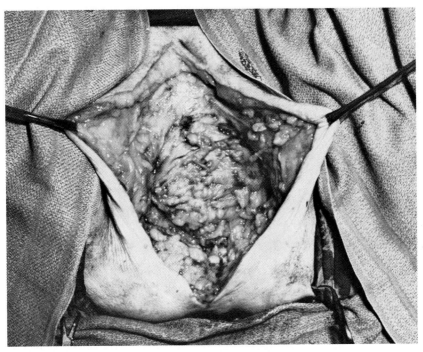

Figure 10-3 Results after imbrication of the hernial sac. (From Ego-Aguirre, E., Spratt, J. S., Jr., Butcher, H. R., Jr., and Bricker, E. M.: Repair of perineal hernias developing subsequent to pelvic exenteration. Ann. Surg., *159*:66, 1964.)

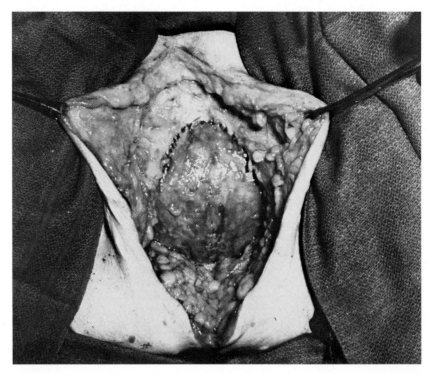

Figure 10–4   Free fascia lata graft in place. (From Ego-Aguirre, E., Spratt, J. S., Jr., Butcher, H. R., Jr., and Bricker, E. M.: Repair of perineal hernias developing subsequent to pelvic exenteration. Ann. Surg., *159*:66, 1964.)

complications among nine cases were attributable to intestinal perforations. As Ego-Aguirre et al. stated,

This surgical repair represents a major undertaking. The danger of injury to intestines intimately adherent to pelvic skin and lateral pelvic wall is a major source of operative risk. In this series, wound infection was associated with recurrence of the perineal herniation. The method of repairing pelvic herniations was successful in five of nine patients (Ego-Aguirre).

REFERENCES

Ego-Aguirre, E., Spratt, J. S., Jr., Butcher, H. R., Jr., and Bricker, E. M.: Repair of perineal hernias developing subsequent to pelvic exenteration. Ann. Surg., *159*:66, 1964.

Kiselow, M., Butcher, H. R., Jr., and Bricker, E. M.: Results of the radical surgical treatment of advanced pelvic cancer: a fifteen-year study. Ann. Surg., *166*:428, 1967.

Appendix 1

The Life Table (Actuarial Survival)

R. LEDUC, M.A.

The purpose of this appendix is to describe the actuarial method used in calculating all end results reported in the tables in this monograph. Every case was followed either to the time the life tables were calculated or to the death of the host. Seventy-five per cent of the cases reported from EFSCH were referred from the Missouri county in which they were born. The Barnes cases are from a broader geographic base. The basic methods were previously described by F. R.

Table A-1   Post-Diagnosis Survival of 195 Bladder Cancer Patients with Transitional Cell Carcinoma (1940–1969)*

1	2	3	4	5	6	7	8
YEARS	No. AT RISK	No. DYING	No. WITH-DRAWN ALIVE	PER CENT SURVIVAL (ANNUAL)	PER CENT SURVIVAL (ACCUMU-LATIVE)	NORMAL SURVIVAL	AGE-CORRECTED SURVIVAL
1	195	65	2	66.5	66.5	95	70.3
2	128	30	3	76.3	50.7	89	56.8
3	95	11	2	88.3	44.8	84	53.3
4	82	6	0	92.7	41.5	79	52.7
5	76	4	5	94.6	39.3	74	52.7
6	67	12	4	81.5	32.0	69	46.5
7	51	8	5	83.5	26.7	64	41.7
8	38	10	2	73.0	19.5	60	32.8
9	26	3	3	87.8	17.1	55	31.1
10	20	3	0	85.0	14.6	51	28.6

*Long, R. T. L., Grummon, R. A., Spratt, J. S., Jr., and Perez-Mesa, C.: Carcinoma of the urinary bladder (comparison with radical, simple and partial cystectomy and intravesical formalin). Cancer, 29:98, 1972.

157

Table A–2 Augmented Working Life Table

TIME	NO. AT RISK	WITHDRAWN ALIVE	EFFECTIVE NO. EXPOSED	DEAD IN INTERVAL	PROPORTION DYING	PROPORTION SURVIVING	ACCUMULATIVE SURVIVAL RATE	σ OF ACCUMULATIVE SURVIVAL RATE	EXPECTED SURVIVAL RATE	AGE-CORRECTED SURVIVAL RATE
1	2	3	4	5	6	7	8	9	10	11
0–1	195	2	194.0	65	0.335	0.665	0.665	0.0339	0.95	0.703
1–2	128	3	126.5	30	0.237	0.763	0.507	0.0361	0.89	0.568
2–3	95	2	94.0	11	0.117	0.883	0.448	0.0360	0.84	0.533
3–4	82	0	82.0	6	0.073	0.927	0.415	0.0358	0.79	0.527
4–5	76	5	73.5	4	0.054	0.946	0.393	0.0356	0.74	0.527
5–6	67	4	65.0	12	0.185	0.815	0.320	0.0346	0.69	0.465
6–7	51	5	48.5	8	0.165	0.835	0.267	0.0336	0.64	0.417
7–8	38	2	37.0	10	0.270	0.730	0.195	0.0313	0.60	0.328
8–9	26	3	24.5	3	0.122	0.878	0.171	0.0304	0.55	0.311
9–10	20	0	20.0	3	0.150	0.850	0.146	0.0292	0.51	0.286

Watson, Ph.D. in another monograph in this series, *Major Problems in Clinical Surgery* (Spratt).

The life table method for comparing end results of different groups of patients has been employed extensively in the past. The life table method yields information on the probability that a patient will survive for a given period of time.

A life table is designed to compute the proportion of patients surviving after given intervals of time, generally one year. It is not necessary that 12-month intervals be used, and when the average survival time is relatively short, intervals as short as a single day may be more appropriate and informative. For instance, in compiling a life table for a cancer site that kills 95 per cent of its patients within two years, shorter intervals would be more meaningful. If all patients in the group being compared have died – so that survival times are available for all – it is probably best to use students to compare the results, but a life table is usually more desirable in making comparisons with groups still having survivors. An example of a life table is given in Table A–1.

In general, groups of patients being studied will still have survivors, and the individual patients have usually been followed for different periods. Obviously, survivors who have been followed for only two years at the termination of the follow-up period yield no information for the life table beyond two years and are "withdrawn" from the life table at this time.

For ease in computation, an augmented working life table is presented in Table A–2.

Key to Numbers Used in Table A–2

COLUMN	EXPLANATION
1	Time interval for all entries in the row
2	Number of patients alive at beginning of interval
3	Number of patients withdrawn during interval (can also include those lost to follow-up, but follow-up was complete on all cases reported in this monograph)
4	Column 2 minus 1/2 column 3: effective number of patients exposed
5	Number of patients who died during time interval.
6	Column 5 divided by column 4; proportion dying during interval
7	1.0 minus column 6: proportion surviving during interval
8	Product of all entries in column 7 to and including this line: cumulative survival rate through given interval
9	Standard deviation of accumulative survival rate
10	Observed survival rate (proportion); survival rate of general populace by age (these rates obtained from Missouri State Life Tables 1949–1951 and 1959–1961; U.S. Dept. of HEW Public Health Service)
11	Cumulative survival rate corrected for age; column 8 divided by column 10

The cumulative survival rate, column 8, indicates the proportion of persons expected to survive a given time interval after some starting point (in this case the time of diagnosis of bladder cancer). For example, of the 195 patients having transitional cell carcinoma, 76 of them survived intervals of four years, that is, they are still living at the beginning of the fifth year interval. Patients are withdrawn alive at the limit of their follow-up period. The method of computing the cumulative survival rate takes this into account.

The standard deviation (σ) of the proportion surviving is given in column 9. If the number of persons in the group is large, one may be relatively certain (95 times out of 100) that the true cumulative survival rate lies between the computed cumulative survival rate and $\pm 2\sigma$. For example, it is 95 per cent certain that the true five-year survival rate is 0.393 ± 0.071, or between 0.322 and 0.464. Stated in terms of percentages, it may be said that between 32.2 per cent and 46.4 per cent of the patients are expected to survive five years.

REFERENCES

Long, R. T. L., Grummon, R. A., Spratt, J. S., Jr., and Perez-Mesa, C.: Carcinoma of the urinary bladder (comparison with radical, simple and partial cystectomy and intravesical formalin). Cancer, 29:98, 1972.

Missouri State Life Tables: 1949–1951 and 1959–1961; U. S. Department of Health, Education, and Welfare, Public Health Service. Volume 2, No. 26.

Watson, F. R.: Statistical methods in cancer research. *In* Spratt, J. S., Jr., and Donegan, W. L.: Cancer of the Breast. Philadelphia, W. B. Saunders Company, 1967, pp. 273 and 298.

What You Should Know about Surgery

BONNIE GARRETT, M.S.P.H.*

Your doctors have decided you will need an operation. Many questions you have about surgery will be answered in this booklet. If you have any further questions, the nurses on your floor or a social worker will be happy to help you.

GENERAL INFORMATION

The surgery suite is on the hospital's sixth floor. All the people who work in surgery, including your doctor, wear green uniforms, caps and masks.

Operations are scheduled throughout the day to keep each operating room busy. If an operation is cancelled or takes less time than expected, there is "open time" on the surgery schedule. For this reason, patients are sometimes scheduled for surgery as *alternates*. If there is "open time," the alternate is taken to surgery. If there is *no* "open time," the alternate's operation will be cancelled for that day.

GETTING READY FOR SURGERY

For a few days before your operation try to eat all the foods and drink all the liquids on your meal trays plus about two extra pitchers of

*Health education at EFSCH-CRC. This appendix was edited by Linda Salfen, B. J., community relations director at EFSCH-CRC.

water each day. This will help your body build strength for your operation with a good balance of fluids and nourishing solids.

It is important for you to learn and use deep breathing exercises before surgery. If done properly, these exercises will make it easier for you to breathe after your operation and will help prevent pneumonia. If you smoke, please *stop* during the days before your operation to improve your breathing and coughing ability.

Practicing some exercises before the operation will make it easier for you after surgery. Remember, after your operation you will have an incision which will make coughing and moving more difficult. The nurses will remind you and help you with these things, but you need to know what to do.

Exercise 1

Roll over in bed frequently. Rolling "like a log," using your stomach muscles as little as possible, will be easiest for you after your operation.

Exercise 2

Move and bend your legs often.

Exercise 3

Take in very deep breaths (so your stomach puffs out) and then *cough* your breath out. Holding a pillow firmly against your stomach will make coughing easier after your operation.

THE NIGHT BEFORE YOUR OPERATION

Your surgery will be scheduled by 3 P.M. the day before. Your doctor will explain the operation, and the nurses will help answer any questions you may have. The *anesthetist* (a specially trained nurse who will give you an anesthetic to take away your sense of pain during the operation) will visit you in the afternoon.

One of the nurses on your floor will bring you the permit for surgery. Before you sign, please be sure to read it or ask a nurse to read it for you.

A nurse will give or ask you to take a pre-surgery bath, which may include special scrubbing of the area where your operation will be done. You may need to take castor oil and several enemas to prepare your bowels for surgery. You may also be given special medication to help you relax and get a good night's sleep.

At midnight a nurse will remove your water pitcher and glass. Please do not eat or drink anything after this time.

THE MORNING OF YOUR OPERATION

Approximately one hour before you go to the operating room, a nurse will give you another relaxing medication. This may also make your mouth dry.

A nurse or an *orderly* (a male hospital attendant) from surgery will take you to the operating room on a stretcher. Remember, he will be wearing the green uniform and cap and perhaps a mask.

As you enter the surgery suite, a nurse will greet you and check your arm band with the name on the chart. She will also ask you your name. This is for routine identification. You will then be taken into the operating room where you will be asked to move from the stretcher to a table.

If you are a woman, a nurse will shave the area where the operation is to be done. If you are a man, an orderly will do this for you. Shaving is necessary to keep hair from contaminating the operation.

A nurse may insert a slender tube in your bladder to draw off urine during your operation. This is called *catheterizing*. It may be done before you go to the operating room. A nurse may also insert a slender tube through your nose into your stomach.

You will not be given the anesthetic until your doctor arrives. We use three types of anesthetic to take away the sense of feeling, or pain. Your doctor and the anesthetist will decide which is best for your operation.

A *local* anesthetic affects only one part of your body. The doctor will inject it into that particular part.

A *spinal* anesthetic affects your body from approximately the waist down, but you will not be asleep. The anesthetist will inject the anesthetic into the space around your spinal cord.

A *general* anesthetic will put you to sleep. You will receive it through an injection into your veins or through a mask.

Feel free to ask questions about your operation at any time.

AFTER YOUR OPERATION

If you are given a local anesthetic, you will be taken back to your room after your operation is finished. The numbness will wear off within a few hours. If you are given a spinal anesthetic, you *may be* taken to the recovery room on the 4th floor.

If you are given a general anesthetic, you *will be* taken to the recovery room. There you receive close and constant care for the first several hours after your operation. The nurse in the recovery room will ask you to cough, turn and breathe correctly as you practiced before going to surgery. She needs your cooperation at all times. Later you will be moved from the recovery room into a regular room, which may not be the same room you were in before, but you will have the same bedside chest and furniture.

After your operation you will be sleepy and will have some discomfort. Tell the nurse if you have pain; she can give you medication for it. If you have any trouble urinating or moving your bowels, be sure to tell your doctor or the nurse.

Your doctor will talk with *your family* about your operation. They will be allowed to see you for a short period of time as soon as your doctor thinks you are ready for visitors. Your doctor will see *you* again on his rounds. He will answer any questions you have at that time.

It is expected that you will be more uncomfortable the second day after your operation than on the day of surgery. Please request your pain medicine whenever you think you need it. You will probably receive your nourishment by vein immediately following surgery. Your doctor will let you know when you may start more activity and when you may eat a regular diet. Continue your deep breathing exercises for about five days after surgery.

The nurses on your floor will help you with any special exercises required following your surgery. They will also give you any special instructions you will need to care for yourself after you go home.

Stitches may be either taken out before you leave the hospital or left in for your doctor at home to remove.

Patient Instructions for Ileostomy and Ileal Bladder Appliance

I. General information
   A. The ileostomy bag is used for patients who have had an operation resulting in urine or contents from the small intestine draining from an opening in the abdominal wall. This opening is called a stoma and is almost always located on the right side of the abdomen.
   B. Some surgeons make a standard ileostomy stoma which will fit a standard bag kept in stock at the hospital. Occasionally a stoma may require a special size or shape attachment. In such cases, the doctor measures the stoma, and the bag is ordered to fit the special requirements. The measurement and the patient's name are kept on record by the company manufacturing the bags for ease in reordering.
   C. The patient or a responsible person who will care for or assist him is taught to apply, remove and care for the bag while he is in the hospital. The instructions should be carefully followed after leaving the hospital.
   D. The patient is supplied with an ileostomy bag set while in the hospital, and he takes this home with him. This set consists of
      2 ileostomy appliances (bags)
      2 soft white belts
      1 spring spreader
      1 dozen special white rubber bands (unless it is a valve set for urinary ileostomy)
      3 tubes of surgical cement
      1 quart of surgical cement solvent
   E. With proper care, two bags (a set) will last approximately six months.

165

II. Replacement
    A. Patients receiving Medicare or Medicaid may obtain re-
        placements through the hospital at no cost. Reordering
        must first be cleared through the social service depart-
        ment in the hospital for eligibility. Then the order is
        placed by the nursing service department and will be
        sent directly to the patient's home address.
    B. Patients ineligible for Medicare or Medicaid may order
        replacements as needed directly from the manufacturer.
        A complete catalogue and price list of appliances and
        accessories may be obtained by writing directly to the
        manufacturer. It is suggested that patients make this
        contact early and decide on the supplies they may need.
        Different manufacturers differ in some of the details of
        appliance manufacture. As the patient becomes ac-
        customed to and adept in managing his ileostomy, he be-
        comes better able to try different appliances and ac-
        cessories to find which is best suited for his particular
        needs. However, until the patient becomes quite expert,
        he should not change from the equipment he was taught
        to manage before discharge from the hospital. The fol-
        lowing is a list of some of the companies which manu-
        facture ileostomy and colostomy equipment:

Atlantic Surgical Company
2287 Babylon Turnpike
Merrick, Long Island, New York   11566

Davol Rubber Company
Surgical Appliance Department
Providence, Rhode Island   02901

John F. Greer Company
5335 College Avenue
Oakland, California   94618

Gricks, Inc.
202–11 Jamaica Avenue
Hollis, New York   11423

Gundrun Frederiksen Company
P.O. Box 481
Oakland, California   94604

Hollister, Inc.
211 East Chicago Avenue
Chicago, Illinois   60611

Marlen Manufacturing and Development Company
5150 Richmond Road
Bedford, Ohio   44014

Marsan Manufacturing Company
5924 South Pulaski Road
Chicago, Illinois   60629

Perma Type Company, Inc.
P.O. Box 175
Farmington, Connecticut   06032

Perry Products
3803 East Lake Street
Minneapolis, Minnesota   55406

The Torbot Company
1185 Jefferson Boulevard
Warwick, Rhode Island   02886

United Surgical Supplies Company, Inc.
11775 Starkey Road
Largo, Florida   33540

The cost varies from approximately $29.50 to $36.50 for each set.
C. The medical, nursing and social service staff will be happy to assist with any problems.
III. Removal of the bag
A. When the bag starts loosening or leaking it should be removed and a clean one applied. Do not leave same bag on more than seven days.
B. Equipment required for removal
1. Cement solvent
2. Cotton ball, applicator, tissue and/or medicine dropper
3. Soap and water
4. Alcohol
C. Procedure for removal
1. Apply cement solvent around loose edge of the bag with cotton ball, applicator, tissue or medicine dropper.
2. Peel disc off gently as solvent is applied.
3. Clean old cement from skin around stoma with small amount of solvent followed by 70 per cent isopropyl alcohol.
4. Wash the area around the stoma with soap and water and dry.
5. Place a cotton ball over stoma to absorb urine.

IV. Reapplication of bag
   A. Keep the skin dry by replacing cotton ball as necessary.
   B. Area may be sprayed or painted, using an applicator, with benzoin tincture.
   C. Apply a very thin coat of surgical cement to both the entire disc surface and the area around the stoma equal to the area of the disc.
   D. Apply a second coat of surgical cement to both the disc and the skin around stoma and again allow to dry for one to two minutes.
   E. Carefully apply bag to skin. Be sure the opening of the bag fits perfectly over the stoma.
   F. Apply pressure with fingers over the back side of disc for one minute.
   G. Fasten the belt to hooks on the bag for added protection. As the belt loses its elasticity through wear and washing, shorten belt by cutting off one end and making a new slot for the hook on the bag.
   H. Secure the drainage end of bag by turning up the end, folding lengthwise in quarters and winding around with rubber band. The urinary ileostomy bag is usually fitted with a valve for emptying.

V. Emptying the bag
   A. Remove rubber band from end of bag and allow to drain into toilet or other receptacle.
   B. For a valve type bag, a three-quarter turn of the valve empties the appliance. Return to previous position after emptying.

VI. Care of bag
   A. Cleaning
      1. Wipe surface of disc with cement solvent but do not remove it all—just enough to prevent too thick a buildup.
      2. Wash bag in hot water with any type of soap or detergent. Do not boil. Give extra care to inside, e.g., scrub inside with baby bottle brush.
      3. Rinse well.
      4. Insert spring spreader into outlet to keep inside surfaces apart and hang to dry by the disc opening.
   B. Deodorizing
      1. If bag acquires an odor, submerge in a solution of Clorox and water by using 2 tablespoons Clorox to 1 quart water. Let it soak one to two hours. Rinse and continue with step 4 above. Diluted Clorox will not harm the rubber.

2. The various companies make and sell deodorants, cleansing powder and brushes. However, the above method is satisfactory.

VII. Tips and suggestions

A. A slight burning or itching may be felt immediately after bag is applied. This should subside in about 30 minutes.

B. Skin must be clean and dry before applying cement. *Do not shave skin around stoma.*

C. Karaya Gum powder may be used to control irritation on skin around stoma. Sprinkle it on—a clean salt shaker containing the powder may be used—and blow or fan off all loose powder. Apply cement and bag as usual over this. Or Karaya Gum washers that fit between the disc and skin can be purchased from the manufacturer.

D. Do not allow any moisture or powder to come in contact with the cement or it will lose its adhesiveness.

E. Talcum powder applied to the bag inside and out when dry and not in use preserves the rubber and prevents odor permeation. *Be sure to remove powder from disc* before applying cement.

F. Tincture of benzoin applied to the disc area around the stoma may aid if there is difficulty in getting the appliance to stick. Allow it to dry before applying the cement.

G. If excess cement is left on the skin or bag after it is firmly applied, dust with talcum powder to prevent sticking.

Appendix 4

Patient Instructions for Care of Colostomy

I. What is a colostomy?
  A. A colostomy is an opening formed by a part of the bowel and serves as an artificial anus through which the bowels will empty.
  B. If you have had such an operation, you will be taught to care for yourself before you leave the hospital.
II. Equipment for irrigation
  A. The equipment you will need to care for your colostomy is listed here. This equipment will be obtained for you before you leave the hospital
       1 enema can
       4 feet of tubing
       1 clamp
       1 male urethral catheter (size 18)
       1 Hygeia or Even-Flo nipple
       1 jar petroleum jelly
       1 glass connector
  B. Additional equipment obtained at home: Wash pan, bedpan, large pail, bucket or some type of receptacle into which the stool can be expelled.
  C. Dressings
    1. The nurse on your ward will give you a supply of dressings furnished by the American Cancer Society to take home with you.
    2. You may use a clean square of cloth over the colostomy opening, or you may purchase dressings at your local drug store.
    3. In some counties the local American Cancer Society chapter can supply you with dressings. Ask your physician, public health nurse or county welfare office if the dressings are available in your county. If not, you can write to

170

Missouri Division, Inc.
American Cancer Society
712 East High Street
Jefferson City, Missouri   65101

They will advise you where you can obtain the dressings.

    4. A two-way stretch girdle, an elastic belt or scotch tape may be used to hold the dressings in place.

III. Instructions for irrigation

    A. Irrigate your colostomy every morning, preferably about the same time each day. Best results are obtained if the irrigation is taken while lying down; however, many patients feel it is more convenient to irrigate while in a sitting position.

    B. Use 1 quart of warm water (do not use soap).

    C. Hang enema can approximately 12 inches above the colostomy opening.

    D. Cut a small hole in the tip of the nipple and place the nipple forward on the catheter 6 to 8 inches. The nipple will prevent you from inserting the catheter too far and will also serve as a stopper, thus preventing immediate return flow of the water. The nipple should be held in place in the colostomy opening.

    E. Allow the water to run slowly (about 15 minutes). If you feel a cramp, stop the flow of water until the cramping has subsided. When all the water has run in, remove the catheter.

    F. Allow 30 minutes for water and stool to be expelled.

IV. General instructions

    A. *Do not* wear a colostomy bag.

    B. Avoid all foods and beverages which may produce diarrhea.

    C. *Do not* take a laxative unless specifically ordered by your doctor.

    D. Perfect control should be attained in about two or three months.

Index

173